WATER
WORKOUTS

WATER WORKOUTS

*A Guide to Fitness, Training,
and Performance Enhancement
in the Water*

STEPHEN TARPINIAN

AND

BRIAN J. AWBREY, M.D.

Lyons & Burford, Publishers

Printed in the United States of America

Design and composition by Rohani Design, Edmonds, WA

10 9 8 7 6 5 4 3 2 1

Library of Congress Cataloging-in-Publication Data

Tarpinian, Steve.
      Water workouts: a guide to fitness, training, and performance enhance-
ment in the water / Stephen Tarpinian and Brian J. Awbrey.
      p. cm.
      Includes bibliographical references (p.) and index.
      ISBN 1-55821-396-1 (pbk.)
      1. Aquatic exercises. 2. Aquatic exercises—Therapeutic use.
I. Awbrey, Brian J. II. Title
GV838.53.E94T37 1997
613.7' 16—dc21

                                                                            97-2427
                                                                            CIP

This book and my life are dedicated to the memory of Krikor Hekemian.

— Stephen Tarpinian

To Matthew and Nathan Awbrey; together they are the joy of my life and my reasons to stay in shape.

— Brian Awbrey

Contents

Acknowledgments

I was really struggling with finishing this book. I had written the first draft and could not see what was holding me back. My research was going well, yet I knew there were a few new advancements in the field of aquatic exercise but could not seem to get information on all of them. Luckily I put the project on hold and a few months later received a letter from Dr. Brian Awbrey stating he wanted to work on the project with me. We met and immediately I realized we would make a great team together. I want to thank Brian for his knowledge of aquatic exercise and for his passion in always improving the techniques and equipment available. Anja Schmidt has been more than an excellent editor and has helped with all aspects of publishing this work and my previous book, *The Essential Swimmer*. And thanks to my favorite running partner, Josephine Piccinic, for being an inspiration in her recovery from her accident and her use of aquatic exercise to aid in that recovery.

— Stephen Tarpinian

I want to thank Steve for searching me out. Special thanks go to Kipp Dye, an accomplished athlete and leader in the field of aquatic exercise who is always eager to pursue advances in aquatic training. I thank Ted Lorenzetti and Milton Velinsky for their creative support and their fervent belief that aquatic exercise and aquatic training are only in their infancy. Finally, I thank Francine Wilson and Mariann Sampson for their assistance in the preparation of the manuscript.

— Brian J. Awbrey, M.D.

Preface

For a fitness consultant and health enthusiast few things are more fulfilling than sharing information that can help heal people and make them feel healthier and more vibrant. I love working with people in the water whether for swimming, deep-water running, or aqua exercise. The water never fails me; it always produces smiles at the end of a session.

This book is designed for anyone wanting to utilize the wonderful properties and environment of water for rehabilitation, fitness, and/or competitive-enhancement exercise. There are some people who simply love the water environment, and therefore, exercising in it makes the most sense for them. There are some people who are limited by an injury, arthritis, or obesity and water provides the healing and supportive properties they require. Lastly, there are athletes and active people looking to add some variety to their cross-training program.

What initially lead me to water workouts was my interest in swimming and love of the water. It was not until I suffered a running injury that I fully realized there were also other forms of aquatic exercise. Quite frankly, like most people, and especially any serious athlete, I thought that any exercise in a pool besides swimming was wimpy. My shinsplint injury ended up being a blessing in disguise by opening my eyes to the limitless ways to exercise in the water. I also saw that the healing properties of water could be enjoyed by everyone, not only swimmers. Further, I discovered the unique properties of water training that can improve my level of fitness.

Water workouts are fast becoming one of the most popular forms of exercise as a result of the low- to no-impact property of training in the water. There are many challenging and enjoyable ways to get a workout in the pool. Virtually every exercise done on land can be taken to the water (yes, I agree, push-ups are a little strange underwater, but I'll explain that later). In the future, we will no doubt be seeing complete underwater gyms for training and rehabilitation. There are fitness centers and clinics right now that have underwater treadmills, poolside water-workout stations, bicycles, and a myriad of handheld equipment—all aiming to fully exploit the therapeutic and resistive properties of water.

In this book we have decided to speak in the first person. When you read "I," it truly represents both of us speaking with one voice. We have written this book *together*, and we bring our unique training and experience to you with our combined enthusiasm and knowledge. This book is broken into eight chapters: the power of water, how to set up a program, aqua aerobics (and move-ment exercises), deep-water running, swimming, water strength-training, sport-specific training, and a training supplement on heart-rate monitoring, flexibility, strength, nutrition, and breathing. The main benefits of each form of exercise are explored, as well as the technique and train-ing principles associated with each. We will also give you a no-frills guide to which pieces of equipment are helpful and which simply fill up your locker and empty your wallet.

1

◎ ◎ ◎

The Power of Water

*Ponce de León spent his entire life searching for
the Fountain of Youth; he would have stayed younger
and lived longer had he exercised in water!*

orking out in the water is becoming extremely popular. It was only a few years ago that people rarely used a pool for anything other than swimming and lounging. These days swimmers are experiencing more and more intrusions on their pool time and space by others wanting to utilize the pool for many exciting new forms of water workouts. What I like most about water workouts is that they have many of the same benefits as swimming.

Now, you do not have to enjoy swimming, or even be a swimmer for that matter, to enjoy the many great benefits of water workouts. (A word of caution: For obvious safety reasons, always swim or work out in an area supervised by lifeguards. Water, especially open water, is an environment for which you always need to have some healthy respect. Remember: safety first.) Swimming can be a lonely activity and for some that is heaven and for others hell. Water workouts are the complete opposite in terms of allowing participants the ability to look around, be social, and utilize music.

INJURY-FREE AND HEALING POWERS

Unlike running or jogging, water workouts are almost injury-free: Any injury is usually a result of poor technique. There is no pounding of the body in the water; all of the movements in the pool are cushioned by the water. Many people, including world-class athletes, have used the healing properties of water to recover successfully from injuries. It is truly an activity for all ages. Infants, children, teens, adults, senior citizens, elderly, pregnant women, handicapped people, injured people, and arthritis patients are examples of the wide range of participants in this fitness activity. Trainers, therapists, coaches, and doctors have been prescribing water activity more and more because it is both safe and effective. Water workouts may be the only safe and effective fitness activity in the hot climate of the sunbelt. Those persons with high blood pressure or heart conditions who might not be able otherwise to exercise vigorously outdoors find that there is not only a cooling effect, but a beneficial cardiovascular effect to working out in the water.

Water workouts can also provide the solution for weather problems. For example, when it is too hot to train you can still get a terrific workout in the pool. At the other extreme, when it is too cold, icy, snowy, or rainy, a water workout is safe and effective. In Boston I treat at least a dozen runners a year for broken ankles and wrists resulting from slips and falls sustained under poor running conditions. The risk of this kind of injury can be prevented by substituting water training on inclement weather days. When in doubt, hit the pool!

For many people, their first introduction to training in water came from the examples of two of America's most popular sports heroes, Bo Jackson and George Brett, whose numerous injuries had been reported in the sports pages of the late 1980s and early 1990s.

FACT: Bo Jackson had suffered a severe hip dislocation that resulted in loss of blood supply to the femoral head and required hip-replacement surgery. During the course of his treatment and recovery he turned to water therapy to build strength and range of motion.

FACT: In the early 1990s, George Brett utilized water exercise to prolong his baseball career by treating sore joints and muscles through sport-specific workouts.

Both Jackson and Brett were introduced to the water in order to heal injuries, and both utilized the power of water to also increase their athletic performance. Since that time their example has led many strength coaches, trainers, and athletes to explore water workouts as a means of improving all-around strength and endurance, as well as sport-specific skills.

It is exactly this kind of publicity that led to an explosion of vertical water exercising in the early 1990s. Vertical water exercise means any type of exercise done while upright, as opposed to swimming exercise, which is done in the horizontal position. In the early 1990s as many as two-hundred thousand people were participating in water workouts, either as a running workout or as an aerobic activity. By 1993 it was estimated that this number had grown to two and one-half million, and in 1995 there were five million regular aquatic exercisers. In the second half of the decade it is estimated that somewhere between ten and twenty million people in the United States and many times that worldwide, will regularly participate in water workouts of one type or another.

TOP TEN WATER-TRAINING MYTHS:

MYTH #1: Working out in the water is a lesser activity than working out on land (i.e., it's wimpy).

REALITY: When Boston Bruins hockey star Cam Neely injured his knee, it was exactly this attitude, that water workouts are inferior to those on land, that led Boston water therapist Kipp Dye to develop a technique using a water running-shoe in conjunction with a cord system. He coined the phrase "elastic-resistive running" to provide a maximally vigorous water workout for professional athletes. Using this system, it has been shown that the exertional intensity of water running can be increased greatly over that of land running. This means that there are ways to work out in the water that are much, much harder than working out on land, while still having all of the benefits of a water workout.

MYTH #2: Water workouts are *not* good for building strong healthy bones (a particular concern for pregnant and postmenopausal women).

REALITY: Medical research has shown that vigorous swimming and serious aquatic activities actually help to build bone calcium, and this is the best way to combat osteoporosis. Regular exercise that pulls at the bones in any direction will lead to increased bone density.[1]

MYTH #3: You cannot build muscular strength from water training.

REALITY: The properties of water lead muscles to actually work harder when moving through water than through air. Because of the increased resistance—and the increased *support* to muscles and bones—aerobic capacity will increase while the risk of stress-related injuries will decrease. Aquatic exercise without equipment offers many cardiovascular benefits. But by adding water-resistance equipment the water workout can be greatly enhanced to increase muscle strength, bone formation, and circulation.

MYTH #4: Water training decreases your libido.

REALITY: Water training actually has a prolonged aphrodisiac effect.[2]

MYTH #5: You must be a good swimmer to utilize water training.

REALITY: Most water-training activities are safe for the novice swimmer and many are performed in shallow water with floatation devices.

MYTH #6: Running in the water is only for rehabilitation and will not aid in performance.

REALITY: Olympian Ed Eyestone did a study of land and water running which showed that the study group with the most land-running speed improvement was the group that trained exclusively in water.[3]

---

[1] Marcus R. Drinkwater, B. Dalsky, G. Dufek, J. Raab, D. Slemend, and C. Snow-Harter, "Osteoporosis and Exercise in Women," Medicine Science in Sport and Exercise, Vol. 24 (6): Supp. 301–07, 1992.

[2] Although there have not been any scientific studies to disprove the myth, the authors challenge you to participate in an aquatics program and prove the reality.

[3] E. Eyestone, "Effects of Water Running and Cycling," master's thesis, Brigham Young University, 1992.

MYTH #7: You cannot lose weight (burn fat) by water training.

REALITY: A water workout can help to keep you in the fat-burning zone. While you may burn more calories on land as a result of the weight-bearing factor, research shows that in water you use a higher percentage of fat as a fuel source.[4]

MYTH #8: Water training does not provide an effective aerobic workout.

REALITY: Not only will your aerobic capacity increase, but your risk of stress-related injuries will decrease.

MYTH #9: Water workouts give no impact to your body.

REALITY: Water workouts in shallow water can provide up to 50 percent of the impact of land exercises. Water instructors recommend use of water-aerobics shoes in shallow water to protect your feet from impact.

MYTH #10: I need a lot of gadgets to get a good workout in the water.

REALITY: While equipment can enhance your workout, the only required item in the water is a swimsuit.

WATER'S PHYSICAL PROPERTIES

Let's take a look at the physical properties of water and find out just why it is superior to air as a medium for exercise. There are three properties that give water the edge: buoyancy, resistance, and refreshment.

Buoyancy Water has a supportive quality that allows you to float. The effects of buoyancy increase as you get into deeper water. If you weigh one hundred fifty pounds on land, you'll weigh fifteen pounds in neck-deep water,

[4] B. W. Evans, K. J. Cureton, and J. W. Pruvis, "Metabolic and Circulatory Responses to Walking and Jogging in Water," *Research Quarterly* 49 (4): 442–49, 1978.

since your weight in water is only 10 percent of that on land. Buoyancy supports the joints and permits movements that might otherwise be limited by an injury. Buoyancy helps postoperative knee, hip, ankle, leg, and back patients to exercise much earlier, and therefore to recover faster and more completely, often improving on prior levels of function. An increase in flexibility is fostered by the increase in range of motion. Lastly, the force of buoyancy gives you a much greater range of motion for all your joints and increased flexibility, allowing you to vary the amount of impact you have on the joints.

Resistance Because water is seven hundred times denser than air and sixty times more viscous, it provides tremendous resistance to movement. This resistance can be slightly greater than on land or many times greater, depending on the speed of your movement. The faster the movement, the more resistance the water offers. Unlike resistance from lifting and lowering a weight on land (which works only one muscle group when you pull against gravity), moving your limb in the water affords resistance in all directions. Exercises performed in water work opposing muscle groups with a single exercise, whereas land exercises can only work one muscle group at a time. When performing a strength exercise on land you perform a positive and a negative movement (the positive lifting against gravity and the negative lowering, resisting gravity). Both use the same muscle. In water, the second movement uses the opposing muscle. This allows water to give a positive-positive training effect. In addition, the combination of hydrostatic pressure and the turbulence caused by movements produce a massaging effect on your muscles. Resistance can be used as a means of water weight-lifting, because hydrostatic pressure (the weight of the water pushing against the body) and turbulence simultaneously stabilize muscles and joints and exert both pressure and a massaging effect.

Refreshment This factor involves many subjective variables, most importantly that of temperature. What feels comfortable and invigorating to one person may be downright hot (or cold) to another. The type of water that you are in is also important. Some people do not mind chlorine while others may feel bothered by it. By experimenting with working out in different kinds of water you can easily discover what feels most comfortable for you. You may find that swimming in the ocean at seventy degrees is great, but stretching in the water requires a trip to the YMCA, where you know they keep the pool temperature at eighty degrees.

The refreshment factor also gives a tremendous massaging effect on muscles and joints. Research studies have shown that exercising in water causes a 10 to 15 percent decrease in heart rate and a 10 percent decrease in blood pressure. This is caused by diminished circulation of blood to the area of the skin, and increased return of blood to the heart and the circulatory system, freeing blood directly to your working muscles. This means that you can get a very good fitness workout for muscles while maintaining a heart rate lower than that possible on land. Heart doctors are realizing this effect, and recommend that all of their patients participate in water training as part of their recovery.

WATER-TRAINING ADVANTAGES AND EFFECTS

Water is a great equalizer. For example, my friend Mike and I can both run as fast as we can in the water while still remaining side-by-side if we use a tether. If we ran as fast as we could on the roads, Mike would soon be in the next county and I would be training alone.

Water workouts allow you to work out every day, yet avoid overtraining. Triathletes know this because they can swim hard every day and not get injured (barring a shoulder injury from poor technique and/or weak shoulder muscles). If they tried this level of effort in cycling or running they would be begging for an injury.

Water allows the body to align properly and works the posterior as well as the anterior muscles. The agonist and antagonist (or the opposing muscles) are worked evenly and the body is developed in a more balanced way. When you exit the water after a water workout you will feel a strong sense of balance and coordination. Contrast this to the wobbly feeling you have after running or performing aerobics on land.

All aquatic workouts have a double training effect: aerobic training (occasionally anaerobic as well) and muscle toning. They are cardiovascular workouts that can use many, if not all, of the major skeletal muscles of the body. In addition to the prime movers (latissimus dorsi, deltoids, biceps, triceps, chest, quadriceps, hamstrings, abdominals, and back), virtually all muscles are employed in a synergistic way. This brings fresh blood and nutrients to all areas in the body. This total body-flushing effect removes dangerous toxins from the body and helps rejuvenate virtually every tissue in the body. Other sports can give you bulky, awkward, and disproportionate muscles. The physique built from aquatic exercise is not only practical but aesthetically pleasing.

Water has an isokinetic training effect that provides equal resistance when you move your joint in flexion and when you move into extension. Therefore, you get two exercises in one. I have coined the phrase "positive-positive training effect" for this phenomenon.

The aquatic environment is very conducive to relaxation and stress relief. Exercising in the water can be a private, introspective activity (swimming laps) or a social activity (participating in an aqua-aerobics class, doing deep-water running, and utilizing a Water Workout Station™ with friends). Track coaches are beginning to water-run their entire team side-by-side as a training method.

HISTORY

Water has been a healing medium since ancient times. Holy water, fountains of youth, and healing hot springs are all examples of aquatic environments that are believed to have special powers.

Water walking and running and water exercise are some of the oldest fitness activities known to man, but it is only recently that they have begun to be tremendously popular. There are ancient Egyptian hieroglyphics and sculptures from 2,000 B.C. showing swimmers and water exercisers. The ancient Greeks and Romans devoted significant time and home additions to their baths.

FACT: Over the past two thousand years very little has changed in the field of aquatic exercise until recently. Elite racehorses are trained almost exclusively in water. To treat the horses' repetitive injuries, trainers run their animals in large swimming pools, well aware of the tremendous benefits of water running and training.

Not only are there scientific advantages to water workouts, it is a fun activity. It is cool in the hot weather, and safer than an icy street in the winter. Many experts have described water workouts as "the high-tech training method of the nineties." We invite you to jump in.

2

⊚ ⊚ ⊚

Designing a Program

We do not plan to fail, we fail to plan.

I wish I did not know this quote intimately. Planning is a process that takes a little discipline. The few minutes you spend devising a plan and periodically revising it will do more for your success than hours in the pool or gym.

The purpose of this chapter is to define the elements of a training program and guide you through designing your own personal program, a program that will give you the results you desire. In this chapter we will explore goals and time management and address the ten concepts of any complete fitness program: aerobic fitness (endurance), anaerobic fitness (speed), flexibility, strength, frequency, interest, volume, duration, rest, and periodization.

TEN CONCEPTS TO UNDERSTAND
FOR YOUR TRAINING PROGRAM

Aerobic fitness: This is the most popular form of healthy exercise, and for good reason. Aerobic activity is any activity that causes your heart rate to elevate for more than twenty minutes. A strong heart is vital to optimum health. The heart rate should not go above the anaerobic threshold (see Chapter 8) or you will go into oxygen debt and have lactic-acid buildup in your muscles. Aerobic fitness is synonymous with aerobic endurance.

Anaerobic fitness: Anaerobic exercise trains your body to break down lactic acid so you can exercise faster for longer periods of time. The fuel for this type of exercise is the sugars in the blood, such as glucose, which only allows for a low-duration, high-intensity workout. This type of vigorous activity is primarily for speed training, but be sure to have a good aerobic base, to prepare the heart and muscles, before attempting anaerobic training.

Flexibility: This allows muscles to stretch and joints to go through normal ranges of motion. Most people do not realize it, but flexibility is one of the gifts of youth. Maintaining, and yes, improving, flexibility keeps us young. In my opinion, flexibility training is the fountain of youth. Water workouts improve flexibility and range of motion by the use of buoyancy, resistance, and the ability of water to support the limbs. Research has shown that running and walking in the water can improve flexibility and range of motion by up to 230 percent.[1] Underwater video recordings revealed that joints have a greatly increased

[1] B. J. Awbrey, "Aqua Therapy: A Proven Combination for Optimal Gamma Strengthening." *Biomechanics* 2(4): 87–9, 1995.

lower extremity range of motion without any conscious effort. Information provided in Chapter 8 will tell you how to improve your flexibility.

Strength: Like flexibility, strength will be improved by your water workouts. Strength-training in water is improved through using various pieces of equipment and through improving the speed and style of water movements. Performing a water workout in conjunction with a workout on land can give a double fitness benefit, as explained in Chapter 8.

Frequency: How often you work out is important. Different activities require different frequencies:

aerobic training—three to six times per week

flexibility—daily

strength—two to three times a week.

Interest: I cannot stress enough that you need to like what you do. There are so many great choices of how to exercise. Here is a short list of some of the activities possible for aerobic training: running (land or water), walking (land or water), aerobics (land or water), kayaking (and rowing), swimming, cycling, cross-country skiing, in-line skating—and the list goes on.

Note that game sports such as tennis, racquetball, basketball, softball, and golf—while healthy activities— are not your best choices for aerobic activity given the random nature of any game-type activity (see Chapter 8 for the explanation). Game sports can be considered *supplemental* to your fitness program.

FACT: Every avid tennis player and golfer that I work with will tell you how much their game improved after they implemented one of our cross-training programs.

All land-based athletes can benefit by cross training and sport-specific training in the water. The effect is one that exercise physiologists call "gamma training," or "gamma loading." This means that certain activities of a sport, such as swinging a bat or boxing, are more difficult to do in water than on land. Therefore, if you can do it well in the water, you will do it in a super fashion while on land. Reduced incidence of injury and improved cardiovascular fitness is welcomed by all athletes.

Volume: A common question is: How much total mileage and/or time should be spent training? This will vary from a total of one hour a week for the beginner to twenty-plus hours for the professional and competitive athlete.

Duration: How long is a workout?

Aerobic: 20 to 60 minutes

Strength: 20 to 30 minutes

Flexibility: 10 to 20 minutes

Rest: As important as workouts, the amount of rest between them is just as important. The rest phase is when the body actually builds muscle and becomes stronger. How much rest do you need? After a difficult or long workout, take a day off or train easy. There are many variables here and stress is probably the major one. Just remember that light exercise always helps to reduce stress. I have found out the hard way that letting stress build up can be very damaging to your health. Reduce or eliminate as much stress as possible, and then put rest in its place. For most exercisers, psychological stress can be even more damaging than physical stress, leading to illness, loss of energy, and erratic sleeping patterns.

Periodization: A method of training in which you alternate hard and easy days, weeks, and months, periodization has proven to be the best approach to training. It prevents burnout and promotes maximum improvement by allowing the body to rest and rebuild after hard training.

OUTLINING A FITNESS PROGRAM

The simple truth: If training is not producing the results you want, and is not enjoyable, you will not do it. Sure, you can use the brute-force method: "I *will* get on that treadmill today! I hate it, but I'll do it anyway!" This method lacks staying power and enthusiasm. For your training program to be successful, it must become part of your lifestyle. Your training should be a part of your day that you look forward to.

There will always be the occasional day when you have to drag yourself to the pool. However, you will have the confidence of knowing how good you will feel afterward, and of knowing that the benefits will far outweigh any resistance you may have to the program. Water workouts are great for keeping you interested because the workouts can be so varied that there is something for everyone to enjoy.

A successful program requires three elements:

1. Specific goals

2. A plan for achieving your goals

3. The discipline to carry out your plan

Follow through on these three elements and you literally cannot lose (well, the fat burning will lead to weight loss). Skip any of these elements or fall short on

In designing a program of training be sure to do exercises that concentrate on all of the major muscle groups of the body. (These are shown below and are referred to specifically in the water-workout chapters and the Glossary at the back of the book.)

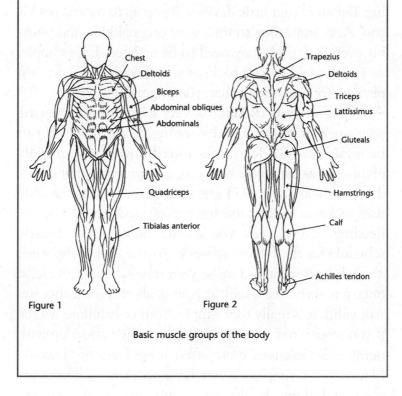

Chest
Deltoids
Biceps
Abdominal obliques
Abdominals

Trapezius
Deltoids
Triceps
Lattissimus
Gluteals

Quadriceps
Hamstrings

Tibialas anterior
Calf

Achilles tendon

Figure 1   Figure 2

Basic muscle groups of the body

designing a program

1 7

your program and the results will be minimal. Seems easy, right? We humans have so many self-sabotage schemes that the process is usually harder than it has to be. Let's take a look at these elements and, in doing so, stack the odds in our favor.

Discipline

I would like to start with the last element: discipline. This is the hardest of the three elements to master because setting goals and making a plan is a one-shot deal. I will give you a little exercise to do in a few pages; you do it, and you're done. Heck, it's even fun to do. Discipline is ongoing. But all of your little devils will pop up to try and outwit you. Also, from time to time your original plan and possibly even your goals may need to be updated. For example, an injury could set you back, or you may find your original plan and/or goals easier than you originally thought.

A log of your training is very helpful for reviewing your workout program and assessing your progress. It can be as simple as a few notes jotted down in your daily planner or as elaborate as a computer program that charts diet and heart rate. Do keep some record—it is the only way to know where you have been and where you are heading. Every week you should make up a realistic schedule for the following week. At the end of the week assess how it went and make your new schedule. At least once a month take a look at your goals and see if they are still valid. It is really that simple. Your only failure will be if you stop. That is pretty comforting. We come up with many great excuses, most often some form of "I would like to but I simply do not have the time." There are some fabulous books on time management (see Appendix I); but it's not the time: It's the commitment. So decide now that your health has a very high priority and schedule your workout time. In your mind make it an appointment you are simply unwilling to cancel. You will be amazed at how you will manage to get more accomplished when your health is at such a high priority.

Specific Goals

It is best to design a program based on the results you would like to produce from your investment (time, energy, money, and creativity) in your workout program. Take a few minutes to fill in the sheet on the next page. It can help tremendously to assess your fitness needs and goals.

This example demonstrates how easy it is to get your goals and the beginning of your fitness plan on paper. You then can put this in a prominent place where you will see it often. Even if you are skeptical, take the 5–10 minutes to do this. I promise it will do more for you than you can imagine. If you do this right you will feel excited and ready to make a plan.

Plan for Achieving Your Goals

With our goals in hand and a clear commitment, we can now devise the plan. That plan is your workouts. If you have the luxury of a coach or a personal trainer, then this chapter will be for your reference only. If, however, you do not and you are going it alone, this section is a step-by-step guide to coaching yourself.

The first question you need to ask yourself is: What do I want from my water-workout program? Some examples of common answers are: to lose weight, improve my running, rehabilitate my injury, learn to swim, exercise my heart. The answer to this question will direct the type, duration, and intensity of your workouts. Here is what I would prescribe for each of these answers.

Lose weight: Unless you have a hypothyroid condition, everyone knows how to and can lose weight. Exercise more and eat less! What a new concept! For eating, you are not exactly on your own, as exercise tends to dampen your

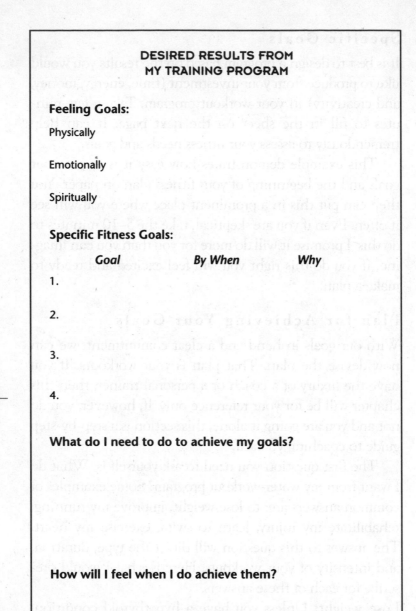

DESIRED RESULTS FROM
MY TRAINING PROGRAM

Feeling Goals:

Physically

Emotionally

Spiritually

Specific Fitness Goals:

	Goal	By When	Why
1.			
2.			
3.			
4.			

What do I need to do to achieve my goals?

How will I feel when I do achieve them?

Here is an example of a filled-in sheet:

EXAMPLE **DESIRED RESULTS FROM**
MY TRAINING PROGRAM

Feeling Goals:

Physically—more energy, stronger and leaner, cure this chronic ankle
   pain
Emotionally—be calm and centered, able to handle anything that
   comes up
Spiritually—connect with who I am and what my purpose in life is

Specific Fitness Goals:

Goal	By When	Why
1. Swim 100 yards under 1:10.	2/1/97	This time signifies being in awesome shape.
2. Complete the local Y 200-lap challenge.	4/15/97	It is something I have never done.
3. Compete in a masters meet.	5/1/97	The thrill of competition.
4. Complete a triathlon. 7/1/97	7/1/97	Triathlon is the epitome of fitness.

What do I need to do to achieve my goals?

—Join masters group, take deep-water running class

—Videotape myself

—Eat better

—Set up my weekly schedule each Sunday evening to allow time for
   workouts.

How will I feel when I do achieve them?

—Unstoppable

---

appetite. And I give you some further help with nutrition (see Chapter 8). For exercise pick a form of aerobic exercise, or better yet, a few different ones (cross training). The key to exercising for weight loss is long duration, high frequency, and proper intensity. You want to be in the aerobic (fat-burning) zone (Chapter 8) for as long as possible. Swim, deep-water run, do aqua aerobics, exercise on the Water Workout Station™—just make sure you have the correct intensity and go for twenty to sixty minutes three to six days a week.

My personal recommendation is to switch every day between water and land exercise, with one day off a week. As you get down to the desired weight, start a strength-training program (Chapter 8). Be patient and make your workout something you look forward to. Even if you can last only two or three minutes the first session, that is fine—simply increase a little at a time. For some the quiet excites them, for others music is an inspiring tool. Use what works for you.

Improve my running: Deep-water running is one of the best-kept secrets for improving your running. It can help in so many ways (see Chapter 4 for specific running techniques and workouts). Swimming and aqua aerobics will help too, if you are inclined to branch out. Just be careful—if you get good at swimming, you may do something crazy like go out and enter a triathlon.

FACT: You get improved performance with water running, and recently this was demonstrated by U.S. Olympic marathoner Ed Eyestone. As part of a master's degree study, he had a number of recreational runners participate in a six-week exercise program in which some ran only in the water, some ran only on land, and some rode a bicycle. At the end of the six weeks, the water runners improved more than either group, improving their land running by 1 percent, or about three to four seconds per mile. They did all of this without running an inch on land for six weeks.[2]

My personal recommendation is to do at least two water sessions a week in addition to your land-based training. Do one easy recovery run after an interval workout, hill workout, or race. This is a thirty- to sixty-minute session, in which you vary your stride length and your intensity (between the low and high ends of your aerobic range, as shown in Chapter 8). The other session should be a speed or interval workout as discussed in Chapter 4. If you are injured, or have a tendency to get injured with increasing mileage, then do your long run in the pool.

Rehabilitate my injury: Almost all movement exercises for injury rehabilitation can get better results in the water. Since there are many different types of injuries, consult with your healthcare provider (M.D., D.O., D.C., or P.T.) for the specific exercises to do, and ask if they can be done in the pool. Take a good aqua aerobics class to help improve circulation and work all your muscles and joints.

My personal recommendation is to get specific movements from your doctor or therapist and then go to the pool and do those. Follow this up with swimming, deep-water running, or aqua aerobics to speed overall recovery and improve cardiovascular fitness.

Learn to swim: If this is your goal then join a good introductory class and get started immediately. When you feel comfortable with your swimming, try using the specific

[2] E. Eyestone. op. cit., p. 5.

technique and training information described in Chapter 5. **Exercise my heart:** My recommendations for this are exactly the same as for weight loss. Interesting, the same plan for maintaining health is the optimum weight-loss program.

When it comes to intensity of aerobic training we can gauge it by heart rate. You can do this subjectively or by taking your pulse. Subjectively we refer to some percentage of perceived maximum. Checking your pulse takes the guesswork out of your training. All the various heart-rate ranges are covered in Chapter 8.

Live by the phrase: "Train, don't strain."

Always listen to your body. Sharp pain anywhere is bad, especially joint pain. Temporary muscular discomfort, on the other hand, is good and should be considered a positive sign that your training is progressing well.

About the only problem with working out in the water is locating a pool that is available at the right time for you. Pools are fairly easy to find in most towns via clubs, YMCA's, and schools. There are reference books to help locate suitable pools (see Appendix I). Don't be limited to pools; use open water like lakes and ponds when appropriate. A suit, goggles, and maybe a cap are the only pieces of equipment that you need. There is, however, some newly developed equipment that increases your training effect, especially in deep water. (See Chapters 3 and 4.)

SUMMARY

Taking a little time to plan before embarking on your new water-workout program is the best investment you can make. If some of these suggestions seem overwhelming, then start out with a small commitment. This is especially helpful if you are just starting to exercise and three to five workouts a week seems impossible. Start at one day a week and evaluate how you feel after that. I have seen many people start with that little commitment, taste the benefits, and increase the number of sessions and duration, effortlessly.

Exercise is one of the cornerstones of what I refer to as the health TRIAD: a sound mind, a fit body (exercise), and a healthy diet. Finding the right balance within these three areas is the art of healthy living.

The beauty is in the balance.

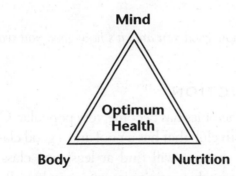

The health triad of mind, body, and nutrition

3

Aqua Aerobics

It's not how good you are, it's how good you work.

INTRODUCTION

Aqua aerobics has become very popoular. Go to any health club that has a pool and a good class schedule, and you will find at least one class of aqua aerobics. Any aerobic activity in water can literally be considered aqua aerobics. Swimming, water polo, deep-water running, and continuously jumping up and down in the shallow end all qualify. Yet usually aqua aerobics refers to those workouts involving a series of movements in the water—whether in the deep (harder) or shallow (easier) end of the pool—that keep the heart rate elevated for a period of time. In this way aqua aerobics is the water equivalent of aerobics classes in the health club, and many classes utilize music as a means of encouragement and motivation. Just as there are many different land-aerobics classes with different emphases (stretch, funk, high-intensity, etc.), aqua-aerobic classes have different areas of focus.

There is one major difference between aqua aerobics and land aerobics—impact. Land aerobics offer both high- and low-impact classes. Most of the injuries in land-aerobics classes come from this impact. In the water, the options are low- and no-impact. This does not mean that aerobics classes are any less intense or any less difficult in water. In fact, I find aerobics classes to be much more difficult in water than on land. The primary reason for this is that you are meeting many times the resistance of land—in three dimensions. Some of the best water-aerobics movements utilize the notion that water resistance and the need to fight buoyancy lead to a better water workout.

As with deep-water running, you get almost all the benefits without any of the overuse injuries associated with land-based workouts. There is important information available to help you get the most out of any aqua-aerobics class you might take, and to allow you to design an aqua-aerobics workout specifically for you. You can even pick your own music to get your motor running. Aqua aerobics are not reserved solely for getting an aerobic workout, but can also be used as a vehicle for rehabilitation from injuries, a method to speed up recovery from difficult workouts, and a way to relax and unwind from a busy day or workout schedule.

THE EQUIPMENT

Although it is not necessary to use equipment for aqua aerobics, there are many different pieces of equipment that are available to enhance a water workout. Most of these make use of the principle that increasing the resistance to your movements increases the intensity of your workout. (Remember: The faster the movement, the more resistance the water offers.) Some equipment can be homemade, like using an empty milk container. In addition to the resistance-increasing type of equipment, a floatation vest, belt, or shorts are needed for deep-water workouts. The buoyancy allows you to do your workout in the deep end with your head above the water, making it a little more strenuous but taking the pressure off your joints. Most classes are held in shallow water at about chest-deep water. The pressure on the joints is significantly reduced in the shallow end, allowing most people, even with injuries, to participate. If the reduced pressure in the shallow end is not enough for you to exercise pain-free, then try working out in deeper water.

Water-aerobics shoes: The notion of wearing shoes in the water may seem silly. However, there are a number of reasons to wear them. Water-aerobics classes can lead to foot injury; those with step aerobics can still have significant impact to the bottom of the foot. Recently, pool directors have been requiring water-aerobics participants to wear shoes to prevent slipping on the pool bottom, injuring the foot, and—an unusual problem—the sluffing off of skin from the bottom of the foot, which plugs pool filters. H$_3$O Works makes the Water Workout Shoe™, which has attachment hooks for elastic resistance cords. Water aerobics shoes range in price from $15.00 to $60.00.

Water Workout Shoe™

Vests, belts, and shorts: These items allow you to do your aqua aerobics in the deep end of the pool. They also help to keep you upright in the shallow end for a water-workout class. An innovative track coach, Glen McWaters, designed a vest for running that he called The Wet Vest™. While The Wet Vest™ is very popular, a drawback to the vest is that for some people the strap between your legs can be uncomfortable. Prices for the vests range from $160.00 to $190.00.

Because of these disadvantages associated with the vest, many types of belts were designed, whose prices range from $15.00 to $60.00. While belts are a less expensive

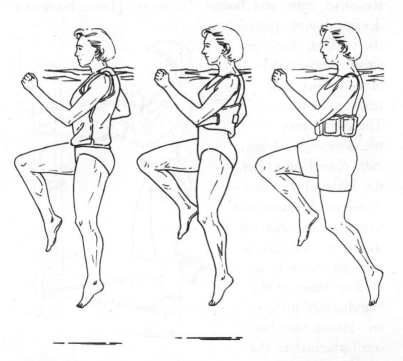

Floatation vest   Floatation belt   Floatation shorts

option, they are plagued with the problem of riding up into the armpits and do not provide the same balance as vests and shorts.

Many problems of the vests and belts have been addressed and overcome by the introduction of Flotation Shorts™. These are neoprene shorts that put pressure on the thighs rather than the crotch. The floatation, which is held on the waist, allows for natural movement in the water. By using the shorts, you can incorporate deep-water running and walking routines, as well as many other types of water exercises, into your workouts. H_2O Works manufactures Water Workout Shorts™, which range in price from $40.00 to $65.00.

Resistive cuffs and boots: These are plastic buoyancy devices that are placed on the ankles, feet, or wrists. Those made of hard plastic may lead to injury. The most versatile devices are foam cuffs placed on either the ankles or the wrists. These are buoyant and have been scientifically shown to increase a workout intensity up to five times. One brand of cuffs utilizes an elastic-resistive cord attached to the poolside to increase

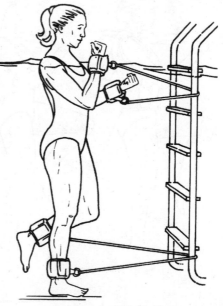

Floatation cuffs and resistive tubing

the intensity of your workout. Prices for H$_2$O Works Water Workout Cuffs™ range from $20.00 to $40.00.

Dumbbells and barbells: These look like ordinary dumbbells and barbells except for the part that would be the weight, which is made of a buoyant material or a plastic paddle. As you move it around underwater, it provides extra resistance to your arm muscles. These devices can also be used to hold you at the surface for back and leg exercises. Many classes utilize empty milk containers (gallon-size) to provide the same effect. You can hold the handle of the container and, with the cap on tight, move the bottle underwater, producing the extra resistance that can make your workout more interesting or at least more intense. When using homemade resistance equipment, be sure to wash out the containers with soap and remove all labels. The dumbbells often have cushioned edges and slip-free grips, and they range in price from $12.00 to $24.00. Barbells range in price from $20.00 to $30.00.

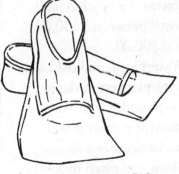

Water dumbbells

Water barbells

Zoomers™ fins

Fins: Especially helpful for deep-water work and swimming, fins make the legs work harder and help with ankle flexibility. I like the Zoomers™ fins best because they are small and work best for swimming, deep-water running, and aqua aerobics. Zoomers cost $35.00 to $40.00.

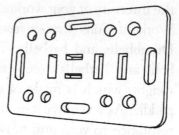

Workout board: This simple, versatile piece of equipment can be used to work both the upper and lower body, and to improve balance and coordination. In addition, this Water Workout Board™ makes a great kickboard. Prices range from $25.00 to $35.00.

Water Workout Board™

Water steps and Water Horse™: As on land, there is an emerging step-aerobics program for the water. A new device called a Water Horse™ combines a step and workout bar together. This allows three-dimensional activities with the arms and is just now being popularized. These are generally purchased by a club and cost between $30.00 and $90.00.

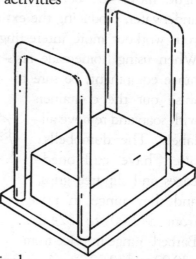

Waterproof radios/cassette players: A device to provide you with music is a must if you are working out alone. Music can often make the difference between a marginal workout and a great workout. Try to use a tape player so that you have control over the music. You can make your own tapes with

Water Horse™
with step

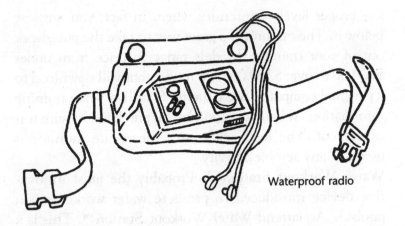

Waterproof radio

slow warm-up and cool-down music, and some high-energy music for the main part of your workout. Prices range from $20.00 to $100.00.

Mitts and gloves:
Resistance of arm movements can be increased by utilizing mitts and gloves with webs between fingers. Mitts and gloves are generally made of a neoprene or soft cloth, and there is a version that uses elastic-resistive cords. These range in price from $15.00 to $25.00.

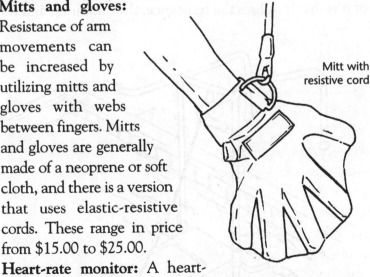

Mitt with resistive cord

Heart-rate monitor: A heart-rate monitor is very helpful for water workouts because it allows you to make sure you are in the right zone. It is very easy to fool yourself into thinking you are working out at the proper level of intensity when, in fact, you are way below it. The monitor is a great way to take the guesswork out of your training. Models range in price from under $100.00 to over $300.00 for a model that will download to a personal computer. See Chapter 8 for heart-rate training information. Whatever monitor you purchase, be sure it is waterproof. The feedback from a heart-rate monitor is useful in any aerobic activity.

Water Workout Station™: Probably the most innovative device introduced to promote water workouts is a poolside Aquatrend Water Workout Station™. This is a stainless-steel exercise machine that actually attaches to the side of the pool, or that sits on a stand inside the pool. The device allows an unlimited number of exercises to be done, just as you might do exercises on land. The beauty of it is that it utilizes the resistance, the buoyancy, and the

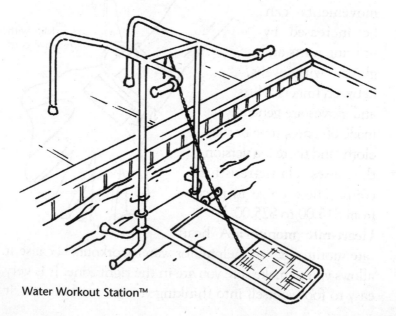

Water Workout Station™

turbulence of water to enhance the workout. The Water Workout Station™ also comes with an optional bicycle, rowing machine, stepper, and Nordic Track™ device, all utilizing the smooth power of water. This station can be a fun and important centerpiece for your water training. The price of the Water Workout Station™ ranges from $250.00 to $695.00.

For help on getting any of these products, check out Appendix IV.

THE MOVEMENTS

There are an infinite number of movements that one can do in the water to make up a combination. In this section we will cover some of the simpler and more common ones.

The best way to get an aqua-aerobics workout is in a class setting with a great teacher. Personal recommendations are usually the best route to finding the best class. Look into your local colleges, health clubs, YMCA, and recreation centers to see what they have to offer. There are even aqua step classes available.

This workout is very similar to the land aerobics class in the studio of a health club. You use the beat of the music to help carry you through the movements. This is the reason for the popularity of aerobics. You get a great workout and feel like you are simply dancing to the music.

The aqua-aerobics workout is made up of a series of movements, each one being repeated several times, followed by a repetition of the complete series. As with all aerobic and anaerobic exercise, you should do a warm-up, a stretch, and a cool-down. The movements you will see here can be used to make your own routine, and/or added to an existing one. See Chapter 2 on "Designing a

Program" for the particulars of structuring your workout for maximum benefit.

TEN ESSENTIAL MOVEMENTS FOR AN AQUA-AEROBICS ROUTINE

Guidelines:

- These movements can be done in shallow or deep water.
- Utilize floatation devices for both shallow and deep water.

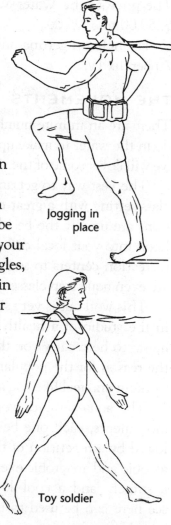

Jogging in place

Toy soldier

1. Jogging in place: Run in place simulating the same running form as for running on land: Relax your shoulders and be sure to keep them down, bring your knees up at ninety-degree angles, and be sure to move your arms in the direction opposite to your legs. There should be no lateral movement. Keep your head erect and looking forward.

2. Toy soldier: This movement is similar to jogging in place except that here you want to keep your legs and arms straight. This movement works the quads and hamstrings a little more thoroughly than jogging does, since the length of the lever is increased in water (because you use the entire leg instead of part of it). This movement can be done in place or by taking long steps.

3. Kick to opposite arm: I like to call this one the cheerleader movement. In this movement you lift your leg to the opposing arm. If keeping the leg straight is too strenuous, try bending at the knee.

Kick to opposite arm

4. Knee-lift kick: Lift your knee up toward your chest and then kick your foot out in front. Alternate legs and keep your hands out to the side or on your hips to help stabilize yourself. This movement works the quadriceps and hamstrings and promotes coordination.

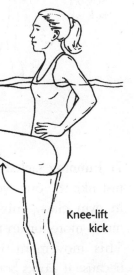

Knee-lift kick

5. Heel kick-up: Lift your foot up behind you, trying to touch your heel to your buttocks.

aqua aerobics

37

Alternate legs and keep your hands out to the side to help stabilize yourself. This movement works the hamstrings and quadriceps and promotes coordination.

Heel kick-up

Scissors kick

6. Scissors kick: Jump straight up and scissor your legs back and forth. Repeat. This movement works the legs and abdominal muscles.

7. Jumping jacks: These are just like the ones you learned in gym class, only they are much more fun in the pool. This movement is great because it works both the upper and lower body.

Jumping jacks

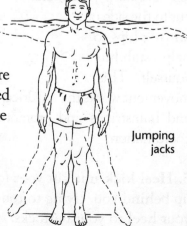

8. Lunges: You need a little room for this one. Lunge forward with your right leg to a ninety-degree angle. Alternate legs. Arms in opposition. This movement gives a good stretch to the psoas muscle.

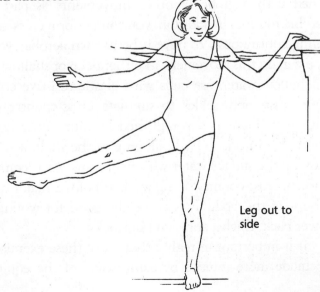

Lunges

9. Leg out to side: Move your leg out to the side as high as you can. Then bring it back down. Alternate legs and use your arms as stabilizers. This movement works the hip abductors and adductors.

Leg out to side

10. Jump forward—jump back: Use both legs to jump forward as though you were playing leapfrog. Then jump back. This is a good movement that really gets the heart pumping since you use both legs together.

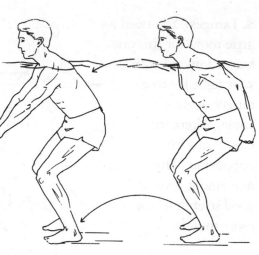

Jump forward—jump back

In addition to the ten essential movements, there is cross-country skiing. Cross-country skiing can be combined with a group of other movements as part of an aerobic routine. In addition, you can perform cross-country skiing continuously to have it be its own aerobic workout. You can do this movement in either deep or shallow water. In shallow water, use cuffs with elastic-resistive cords on your wrists and ankles to simulate cross-country skiing. This movement is accomplished by alternating legs and hands from front to back, lunging in the shallow end and moving the surface water with your arms. As is commonly known, cross-country skiing works all of the major muscles groups of the body. It is especially good for working the lower back, thighs, arms, and buttocks.

It is important to realize that all of these exercises can be made more intense by using some of the equipment described earlier. This would augment the resistance factor of the water, make the exercise more difficult, and improve both muscle strengthening and fat burning. Besides, admit it: We all love pool toys.

All of these movements can also be done in deep water, although they become a little more taxing there. Two more movements that can be done *only* in deep water are vertical kicking and scissors.

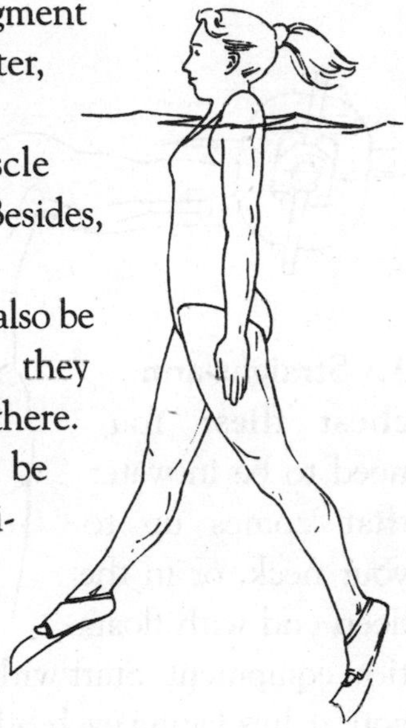

The vertical kick is a flutter kick in the vertical plane. Use fins for added resistance.

Vertical flutter kick

If scissors kick utilizes a scissoring type of movement to work the leg muscles and is enhanced by the addition of ankle cuffs.

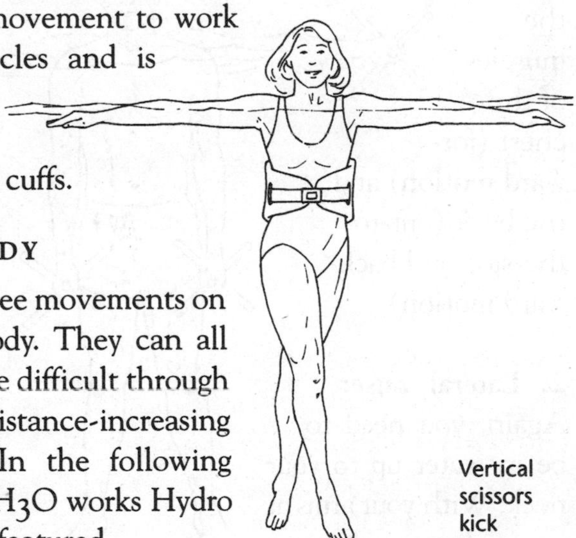

UPPER BODY

There are three movements on the upper body. They can all be made more difficult through the use of resistance-increasing equipment. In the following illustrations H3O works Hydro Paddles™ are featured.

Vertical scissors kick

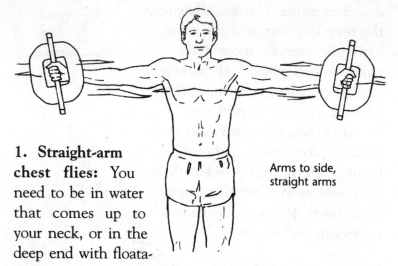

Arms to side, straight arms

Lateral raise

1. Straight-arm chest flies:

You need to be in water that comes up to your neck, or in the deep end with floatation equipment. Start with your arms extended in front of you, palms facing each other. Move both arms to the side and as far back as you can. Then return your arms to the starting position. This movement works the muscles of the chest (forward motion) and the back (out-to-the-side and backward motion).

2. Lateral raise:

Again, you need to be in water up to your neck. With your arms at your side, raise them up

and out to the side (laterally) and
then bring them back down.
This movement works
the shoulders and
arms. Another way to
work the shoulder muscles
is to make a paddle
movement with the
barbell (make sure
it is the pool foam vari-
ety!). With your hands placed
in front of you about two feet
apart, alternately dip the ends
in the water.

Paddle
movement

**3. Biceps curl/Triceps
extension:** Again, you need
to be in water that comes up to
your neck. Start with your arms
out at your side. Bend at
the elbow and bring your
arms up, then bring them
back down to your side.
When you bring your arm
up you are using your
biceps; when you are
moving them down
you are using your
triceps.

Arms to side, bent
elbow

ABDOMINALS AND LOWER BACK

By utilizing the wall, a ladder or the ladder or Water Workout Station™, you can do many additional exercises. Here are two of the more popular ones for the abdominals and lower body:

- **Abdominals:** With your back on the wall, pull your knees to your chest by contracting your abdominals. To work the obliques (the sides of the abdomen), bring your knees up to your shoulder, alternating right and left shoulder.

- **Kicking:** Kick your legs from the same position as described in the abdominal movement. This works all the muscles of the leg. You can do a flutter-type kick or a froglike kick.

Kicking while
at pool wall

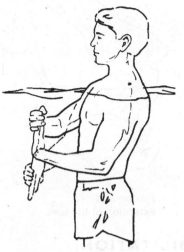

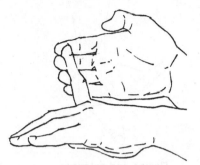

Flexion and extension
of wrist

Flexion and extension
of the fingers

WRIST, HAND, ANKLE, AND FOOT

The wrist, hand, ankle, and foot are complex structures containing a great number of bones and joints, and they are therefore common areas of injury. There are many little movements to help get mobility back in these areas after they are injured. These are lower-intensity movements and are good to do as part of a warm-up and cool-down.

Wrist and hand: Submerge your hand and wrist. Work the wrist by flexing, extending, and moving your hand side-to-side. Then work the individual fingers by flexing and extending each one individually. Use the other hand to assist.

Ankle and foot: Sit on the edge of the pool or on a step. Work the ankle first by flexing, pointing, inverting, and everting the foot. Then work the individual toes by flexing and extending each one individually with your hand.

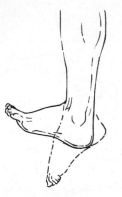
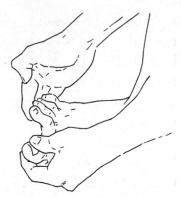

Flexion and extension
of the ankle

Flexion and
extension of the toes

WORKOUTS: REHABILITATION, FITNESS, AND IMPROVED PERFORMANCE

REHABILITATION

Aqua aerobics for rehabilitation is very popular. The support of the water is welcomed by sore and injured muscles, tendons, ligaments, and joints. This is an area where you need to work closely with your physician and/or therapist (for more information, see Appendix II). Ask your health-care providers which movements in this chapter they recommend and what additional specific movements they suggest for your condition. Be sure to ask if there are any exercises or movements which you should *not* do. With this knowledge you can incorporate specific exercises into a class, or you can make up your own routine.

FITNESS

Aqua aerobics for general fitness has a double advantage. You get a total body workout and a recovery workout at the same time. Aqua aerobics is one of the only activities that not only works your muscles for strength and works your heart, but also helps you recover from any land-based training that may be leading you toward an injury. Injury is one of the most common reasons why people drop out of their fitness program, so aqua aerobics is the best addition to all of your land-based workouts—and as a routine of its own. With the knowledge provided in this chapter, it is up to you to find the percentage of water- versus land-training that is optimal for you.

IMPROVED PERFORMANCE

For the professional competitive athlete, and even the serious weekend warrior, aqua aerobics can be used in three ways: as a fun workout to help you recover from hard training, as a sport enhancement, and as a skills or rehabilitation workout.

For a fun workout you can participate in a group class (we have all seen clips of professional football teams taking an aerobics class for flexibility, coordination, and fitness) or simply go solo with or without music. The competitive athlete needs to work specific skills closely with a coach to see which movements can be performed in the water to improve strength, flexibility, and timing. For a rehabilitation workout, you need to focus on the injured area and the movements that help improve range of motion, strength, and endurance.

SUMMARY

Aqua aerobics is an exciting new way of exercising that has mass appeal. Just as deep-water running is the counterpart to land-based running, aqua aerobics is the counterpart to aerobics on land. You can increase the intensity of the workouts by increasing the speed of some of the movements and also by using equipment that adds to the resistance you experience. Let the power of the water work for you by incorporating an aqua-aerobics routine into your regular fitness program.

4

Deep-Water
Running and Walking

*A pioneer who was known for his running speed
asked a Navajo Indian Chief this question: "Who
among your tribe is the fastest?" To which the
Chief replied: "Deep-Water Running."*

INTRODUCTION

I like many others, thought that deep-water running
was reserved for the injured athlete. Many times while
, at the pool for swim-team practice in college, I would
see members of the football, basketball, and track teams
either walking around in the shallow end or donning a
buoyant vest or belt and venturing into the deep end for
some deep-water running or walking. It was only when I
had a stress fracture of my tibia five years ago that I learned
the power of deep-water running, not only for injury prevention and recovery, but also for improved performance.

Although I focus on deep-water running in this chapter, deep-water walking is a wonderful exercise and, essentially, is just a slower-paced version of deep-water running. I have encountered many people who cannot run on land but are able to run in the water. So start out walking and watch how fast you begin to pick up the pace.

FACT: I had been plagued with shin splints for over a year. Nothing seemed to help. I cut back on my running, I got every therapy possible from physical therapists including electrical stimulation, massage, and ice. I tried total rest. I tried running easier, faster, longer, shorter, and on different surfaces. It was not until I combined Aaron Mattes' stretching and strengthening protocol (see Chapter 8) with deep-water running that I cured the problem. My recovery resulted in my competing in the 1993 Hawaii Ironman, including 26.2-mile full marathon run at the end! I am convinced that without the deep-water running and stretching and strengthening, I would not have been in the race.

Some advantages to deep-water running are the ability to train during periods of intense heat; the ability to do extra workouts of running without risking injury; the ability to start a running or fitness program even if you are overweight or injured; and the ability to improve performance. The major advantage behind deep-water running is that you have no gravity to deal with, therefore it is less stressful for joints. Water walking and running has generally been viewed with skepticism by athletes as an inferior exercise tool. The medical facts, however, prove otherwise: Joint motions underwater increase between 100 and 230 percent compared to land walking and running.

Our current knowledge of water-exercise physiology affirms that there is a 10 to 15 percent decrease in heart rate and blood pressure during a running workout in the water. This is extremely helpful for those with hypertension and heart disease, children, the elderly, and pregnant women.

For those interested in improving running performance, a further advantage of deep-water running is improved gamma loading and gamma strengthening. This means that physical training and rehabilitation are carried out harder and faster, and strengthening occurs across greater joint motions in the water.

You should realize that your water work needs at least a minimal amount of supplemental dry-land exercise. Walking or jogging on land and weight training are good examples of the types of exercise to supplement deep-water running. Utilizing various mediums and disciplines for your exercise program is at the heart of cross training. Cross training has proven to be very beneficial to athletes and fitness enthusiasts. I promote a balance between land and water training.

THE EQUIPMENT

Equipment for this activity is optional. (Well, that is not entirely true—most pools do require a swimsuit!) Almost all deep-water runners use some sort of device to help with floatation; most of these aids have been designed specifically for deep-water running. These floatation devices are designed for two tasks: They hold you upright in the water, and they hold your face and mouth above water so that you can breathe normally.

It is possible to run without a floatation device, but quite often a good part of your running stride turns into a swim stroke and you find yourself paddling in order to keep your head above water. Without floatation you will not be able to do an easy recovery run, since high intensity is required for maintaining your body position.

All of this equipment is illustrated and more fully described in Chapter 3. For help in obtaining any of these products, check out Appendix IV.

Vests: These may look like life-preserver jackets, but they are not. Life vests force the wearer to float on his/her back, allowing the head to stay out of the water. The running vest, on the other hand, is designed to float you in a neutral position so you can achieve your running stride. At first the vest may feel cumbersome, but after a while you may not even realize you have it on. If you are not comfortable in a water environment, you should probably go with a vest. One common complaint is that the strap between your legs can be uncomfortable.

Belts: These perform nearly the same function as the vests and do a fairly good job. However, they fail by not fully stabilizing the body and by riding up as you exercise. The belts force you into an awkward flexed position, whereas the vest and floatation shorts keep you in the correct position. The belts are a less expensive option, however.

Shorts: After having used various belts, vests, and shorts, I have found Flotation Shorts™ to perform best. They help keep you in good form and allow for a smooth running stride.

Shoes: Water-exercise shoes protect the foot and prevent slipping on the pool bottom during shallow walking and running. The most innovative water shoes I have used are physical therapist Kipp Dye's WaterWorkout Shoes™. These shoes have built-in rings that allow you to attach a cord to create a very intense running workout.

Tethers: The designers of water-workout equipment have thought not only of making the workout better, but also of the social aspects of running. By the use of either fixed or elastic-resistive tethers, running in the water can be even more of a social activity than on land.

There are two categories of tethering systems:

The first is a simple tether that attaches to the floatation device and simply holds you in place. This is very useful in pools that are small, allowing you only two to three strides before you must stop and turn; and even in larger pools a tether allows you to avoid interfering with other swimmers and runners. Many hotel and home pools that would otherwise be useless can be wonderfully useful with a tethering system. If budget is a consideration then consider making a tethering system yourself by attaching yourself to a rope or something similar. The same tethering system can be used for swimming in small pools.

Elastic-resistive tethers are cords that are attached to shorts, cuffs or shoes and allow you to increase your resistance. By increasing speed and stride length in the water, you increase the resistance and thus the intensity of your workout. A number of collegiate track coaches are using this technique to run their entire track team in the water side-by-side. The fastest runner on the team will always come out ahead.

Resistive cuffs: For most runners, the water provides more than enough resistance. *Want more?* Simply increase the speed of your movement, and the resistance increases as your limb speed increases. *Want even more resistance?* Then try resistive cuffs. A recent scientific study has shown that energy expenditures during a running workout can be increased up to five times through the use of resistive cuffs worn around the ankles. I don't recommend wearing cuffs on the wrists for runners, since cuffs can impair arm swing form. I do recommend them on both ankles and wrists for other water training. *Want the most resistance?* Studies have also shown that the use of elastic-resistive cords on the cuffs (or shoes)—as opposed to a fixed tether—offers the *most* intense water running workout that can be had.

Fins: The fins make the legs work harder and help with ankle flexibility. I like the Zoomer™ fins best because they are small and work best for swimming, deep-water running, and aqua aerobics.

Heart-rate monitor: A heart-rate monitor is essential for deep-water running, since it is easy not to know the level of your training session. The monitor eliminates the guesswork and allows you to quantify your training session. See Chapter 8 for more details on heart-rate monitoring.

Waterproof radio/cassette player: This adds variety and often a tempo to your individualized running program.

FACT: David Brennan of the Houston International Running Center has developed a running program based upon tempo and cadence. He pipes the cadence of a metronome into the training runners' headsets (and heads) so that they reach a desired speed. His associate, Dr. Robert Wilder of Baylor University, has correlated this running cadence in the water with heart rate.

THE TECHNIQUE

The technique for deep-water running, while simple, is easy to perform incorrectly, thus diminishing much of its effectiveness.

THE BASICS

First, remember that you are simulating running on land in the water. Many of my students frequently have trouble getting a fluid stride for the first week or two of practice. Be patient; it is awkward for everyone, and after two or three sessions you will start to feel more comfortable.

BODY POSITION

Your body should be lined up without any bend in the waist. You should have a slight lean forward of only a few degrees; again, no bend at the waist—this is a total-body lean. The position simulates the body's running position when on land.

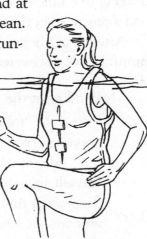

Correct water running position

MOVEMENT

Good running form uses the arms and legs in opposition—the legs line up under the respective hip and the arms stay low and close to the body. Position your hands so your palms face each other slicing through the water. The correct opposition is right leg forward and

Correct arm and hand position while water running

left arm forward, then left leg forward and right arm forward. As each leg and arm is driving forward against the water's resistance, the opposing limb is driving back. There is a natural tendency to take short strides because of the extra resistance of water. Be sure to fully extend your stride. Do not forget to move your arms. Drive the arm back and feel the resistance against your triceps. No doggy-paddle, this is running!

Keep your body aligned, symmetrical, and smooth throughout this alternating movement. Breathing should be smooth and deep, concentrating on the exhale (see Chapter 8). To hold a good body position keep your neck and shoulders relaxed and your abdomen and lower back contracted. Keep that position even if you're tired.

FACT: A University of Georgia study showed that a quarter-mile water walk (440 yards) was more intense than walking one mile on land. Water walking can be intense and is practiced by thousands of older Americans every day.

After many hours of training athletes in deep-water running, I've discovered some common problems:

1. Bending at the waist and leaning forward.

2. Doing the "robot" walk instead of the normal opposition pattern. A robot uses both limbs on one side at the same time. Many people (myself included) do this when they first do deep-water running. If you feel really awkward and are not sure why, check to see if you have this "robot" situation.

3. Dog-paddling with the arms instead of performing the normal opposing movement with arms down and slicing through the water.

4. Keeping arms out to the side instead of elbows in.
5. Bringing arms up too high.
6. Not using your muscles through the entire range of motion. It is very easy to be lazy and to take little strides, not fully engaging your quadriceps (the muscles in the front of the thigh) and hamstrings (the muscles in the back of the thigh).
7. Leaning backward with your legs in front of you almost as though you were riding one of those recumbent bikes at the gym.
8. Having undue stress in the neck and shoulder region, caused by chilly water or by dog-paddling your arms.
9. Not utilizing the ankle joint to flex and point the foot.
10. Breathing too shallowly—not taking long controlled breaths.
11. Using a bicycle-pedaling motion instead of a running stride.

WORKOUTS: REHABILITATION, FITNESS, AND IMPROVED PERFORMANCE

Now that you have the technique mastered (remember, achieving proficiency takes one to two weeks, so be patient), let's look at how to train in your newly developed skill.

One of the really great aspects of deep-water running is that you can simulate virtually every workout that you can do running on land. Everything from an easy walk to intervals can be simulated in the pool. The pool deck may not be as interesting a scenery as the road (well, it depends on who's on the deck!), but you will no doubt feel much fresher after a run in the water than you would with a land workout. You need not work out only in the pool; an open-water area (a calm ocean beach, lake, or bay) can work fine and allow you to be in a nicer environment. If boredom is a problem, try using a waterproof radio or cassette for a little healthy distraction.

There have been many recent advancements that allow the water exerciser several ways of water running, letting you find the one you like best and encouraging variety. Run a few different ways! The most popular is running free, followed in popularity by the use of a tether. It is also possible for you to run stationary while holding a set of underwater bars or the pool ladder. In my opinion, all of these options are better than a treadmill.

Let's look at how different kinds of workouts compare for rehabilitation, fitness, and improved athletic performance.

REHABILITATION

We know that runners suffer an injury rate as high as 20 percent each year. These injury-prone runners have been hitting the pool to do deep-water running with more frequency.

FACT: American record-holder Steve Scott, Olympic marathoner Joan Benoit-Samuelson, and Olympic marathoner Ed Eyestone have spent so much time water running—and like it so much—that we can see them advertising various water-running products.

There is no better way to rehabilitate a running injury than to keep running—but only in the water. Remember that running on land delivers a force of some three to four times your body weight through your bones and joints. This happens with each and every step. In deep water you have no impact, helping you to recover from these injuries.

I advise that you always consult with your physician before participating in any type of aerobic exercise, and especially before you begin a program of rehabilitation. It is always important to have an accurate diagnosis before you begin therapy. If you have been properly evaluated and diagnosed, and are suffering from injuries of the lower extremities or back, you will benefit from a deep-water running program. Deep-water running is indicated for any type of stress fracture, and it can even be performed with a cast cover for those with acute fractures. Water running is especially helpful for athletes with shinsplints; various types of tendinitis of the foot, ankle, and knee; arthritis; Morton's neuroma; and muscular strains. Water therapy is also emerging as an important treatment for the spine. It has been proven to be particularly successful in the period both before and after surgery. Water training allows you to stay fit until the actual surgery, even if you can't exercise on land. After surgery, rehabilitation can start much earlier in the water due to the water's supportive properties. Often, your insurance plan will pay for a water physical therapist to do your initial training.

Why does water running help these conditions? For example, with shinsplints, the primary condition is that of tight calf muscles. By deep-water running, not only do you take the stress off the muscles of the calf, but you increase flexibility and help stimulate the healing of the area involved. It is very important to start treatment immediately if you have shinsplints, since uncorrected shinsplints lead to stress fractures. Take it from someone who has been there. The rehabilitation for stress fractures is usually a minimum of three months, while the rehabilitation for shinsplints can often be only three to six weeks. Deep-water running allows you to have all the benefits of running without the risk of injury.

The increase in your risk of injury when you run on land is directly associated with the amount of mileage you do each week. The majority of these injuries are minor aches and pains and tendinitis, but some can be quite serious. For land running, there is an increase in injuries associated with runners who have logged a number of years—as well as a number of miles.

Many runners benefit greatly from—and learn to love—substituting water running for land running two to three times a week. I mention this only to emphasize that your water work needs at least a minimal amount of supplemental dry-land exercise. Walking or jogging on land and weight training are good examples of the types of exercise to supplement deep-water running.

There is a distinct difference between pain and discomfort in the context of injuries and rehabilitation. Any driving sensation that tightens up your entire body and makes you want to scream is pain. Continuing the movement that causes the pain will just bring on more. The correct thing is to stop the movement immediately. Discomfort, on the other hand, may be a necessary state to go through in order to achieve full recovery. There is stiffness and discomfort with most injuries as you start to use that part of the body in ways that it has not moved in a while. This ability of the body to resist movement insures you the rest you will need in order to let the area heal. Usually the discomfort is felt near the end of recovery and is a good sign that the injury is healing well. Doing light exercise with a little discomfort may be the best medicine. When in doubt, consult your healthcare professional. Do not push through pain. The "no pain, no gain" philosophy can put you in a setback situation. Be patient. The body has a remarkable ability to heal itself: You can assist it by listening to the signals that it gives you.

First things first: Can you walk in deep water with a vest or belt on and have no pain? If so, skip to the next paragraph. If not, then read this paragraph. You need to start out with simple and abbreviated movements in the water, to help promote blood flow and to allow the legs to achieve a natural range of motion (which is much greater in the water than on land). You can begin with something as simple as:

- Gently moving your leg back and forth in the water.
- Gently rotating your ankle.
- Gently flexing and extending the knee or hip.

These movements will have many therapeutic effects including:

- Providing fresh blood to the injured area.
- Invigorating the nerves and muscles that have been dormant.
- The water's movement around the muscle massages the area.
- Increasing flexibility.

- Increasing range of motion.
- Increasing venous return from swollen arms or legs.

Try walking in deep water every other session to see if you can do so without pain. When this is possible, walk at an easy pace for a duration of 5 to 45 minutes, depending on your comfort level. Then try running in the water every other session.

Can you run in the water with no pain? If you have a little pain, you need to continue walking and slowly increasing your pace until running is possible. If you have no pain at all, you can start by simply going at an easy aerobic pace (see Chapter 8 on "Heart-Rate Monitoring"). Concentrate on good form and pick a duration you feel comfortable with. If your injury has kept you inactive for an extended period of time you may start off with as little as five to ten minutes. Train as often as you can (every day is okay with this activity) and add a minute or two every session until you reach thirty minutes. When you've reached this goal, you are ready to start doing some more intensive workouts. See the workouts in the sections on "Deep-Water Running for Fitness" or "Improved Performance" that follow in this chapter for detailed workout information.

Consult your physician or therapist as you progress and integrate your training on land with your water training. I strongly encourage you to continue your water training even after the injury is completely healed. Water training can be one of the best ways to stay healthy and avoid overtraining injuries. In addition to rehabilitating the injury, you get the added benefit of working on your aerobic fitness.

What can you do if an injury is preventing you from running, or even standing, on land? Many experts in the field of water rehabilitation recommend that you follow a progressive program of weight-bearing activity in the water. **FACT:** Boston-based rehabilitation experts Igor Burdenko and Kipp Dye would recommend that you first start in very deep water with gentle and controlled movements, doing movements that do not cause pain. Then you can progress from deep water to shallow water. Then from shallow water to controlled conditions on land and on to increasing activities on land, supplemented with water workouts.

DEEP-WATER RUNNING FOR FITNESS

The analogy that can be made here is that deep-water running for general fitness is like jogging. Generally, people who run for fitness and not competition refer to what they do as jogging. Basically, it is lower-intensity running. There are many reasons why one would run for fitness:

- Lose or maintain weight.
- Improve cardiovascular endurance.
- Remove toxins from the system.
- Improve circulation.
- Improve energy for mental clarity and an elevated mood.

These are the same reasons cited by most people for any fitness program, regardless of the particular discipline or disciplines (cross training) of choice.

Most people start up an exercise program for the first two reasons: weight (loss and maintenance) and cardiac health. For these reasons, and for all the other benefits of exercise, the intensity and duration need to be measured accurately. It is not enough to simply say: "Yeah, I went about twenty minutes at a good clip." As a coach, I could live with the twenty minutes, but a good clip? What does that mean?

Intensity in aerobic training can be accurately measured by your heart rate. This is why it is important to measure your heart rate either by taking your pulse or, preferably, by using a heart-rate monitor. See Chapter 8 on "Heart-Rate Monitoring" for specifics on intensity ranges.

I like to view everyone that I work with as an athlete. Therefore, the workout for a competing athlete and a fitness enthusiast are not very different. Most of the difference is in the volume of work that you do. For example, a competing 10K runner may spend as much as twelve hours a week running, whereas a fitness runner will spend one to three hours per week running. Also, the fitness runner focuses on the steady-intensity work with little to no anaerobic training.

Once the optimal training heart rate is established, it is simply a matter of warming up for five to ten minutes before getting in the "zone" for twenty to sixty minutes, and cooling down for five to ten minutes. This regimen should be followed three to five times per week. To keep things interesting, you can alternate between long and short strides and move your intensity from the low end of your zone to the upper end.

IMPROVED PERFORMANCE

This section is for the competing athlete, whether you are a runner, triathlete, or just a training junkie. Here I will lay out the different types of workouts to help improve your fitness to the highest level of speed and endurance. For the competing athlete, and realistically for all, deep-water running needs to be integrated with running on land.

The greatest gain to the competitive runner is the ability to train more (in time and intensity) yet at the same time reducing the risk of injury. As I mentioned before, one of the terrific benefits of deep-water running is that you can simulate almost all the same workouts that are done on land. "Hill repeats" is a difficult workout to simulate accurately, although, inasmuch as hill repeats are a form of interval training, they can still be done. First, let's look at the different types of workouts and then at how we would put them together to make a workout program.

Long easy distance: Many coaches refer to this as long slow distance, although I have found the word slow is not accurate. The key is *effort*, and that should be easy. Psychologically, it makes no sense to ever think of anything you do as slow. Many competing runners are realizing that doing the long run in the water really makes a difference. Instead of that "dead leg" feeling after a long run on land, and the possible overuse injury, you end up feeling rejuvenated after running in the water. In addition, the run can be longer if desired.

FACT: Top professional triathlete (1995 Canada Ironman Champion) Michael McCormack runs as long as three hours in the water for his long run every week. If he consistently ran that long on land, he would never make it to the starting line.

Objective: The main goal here is to go at an easy aerobic pace for a long period of time. This accomplishes three things. First, you train your fat-burning system—the fuel of choice for endurance athletes due to its near limitless availability. Second, you build endurance. Third, you build confidence that you can go the distance.

How it is done: Definitely monitor your heart rate and try to run for at least the time of your race. If you are a 5K or 10K runner, run longer than the expected finish time. For a marathoner, run for as long as you will in the race. Always be conscious of technique; it is easy to fall into bad habits and lose some of the effectiveness of the workout, especially in this distance workout. Vary the intensity within your aerobic range (see Chapter 8) and change stride length and frequency from time to time. Unlike on land, where you need to be concerned that going too long may injure you, in the water you can go longer with only the fear of losing spouse, children, and/or friends when you stay at the pool for four hours every Sunday.

Frequency: Once per week.

Recovery: This run is meant to be an easy aerobic session to allow your body to become stronger from hard sessions, whether they are on land or water. Due to the therapeutic effects of the water, recovery in deep-water running can actually be a little more intense than on land. I have found that the muscles actually recover better with a little increased intensity. It is actually possible to go hard almost every day in the pool (something you would not dream of on land). This is the power of water.

FACT: Many successful elite runners use the water strictly for recovery or to get in a second run of the day. Mike Powell, Olympic gold medalist and world-record holder in the long jump, does recovery runs in the water daily.

Objective: To continue to work on endurance recovery, yet allow the body to repair tired and sore muscles. Recovery runs also allow the mind to rest from the intensity of hard training sessions.

How it is done: There are many ways to do this run. The key is to keep the intensity on the low side of the aerobic range (see Chapter 8), or even slightly under the range. Alternate between long easy strides and short quicker ones. Duration can be as little or as long as you like.

Frequency: The day after any hard effort is ideal (or even the same day right after the hard effort). Two to three times per week.

Interval training: This is the cornerstone of any serious runner's training program. Interval training is the part of your training in which the intensity is the highest. This form of training develops speed and power and builds endurance. One paradox of running is that you need quality interval training to improve; however, interval training increases your risk of running injuries. The demands of interval training on the body are great, and that is why many of the running injuries we see are related to intervals.

Almost all coaches require at least one day of rest between interval sessions; some coaches recommend only one interval workout (sometimes referred to as speed workout) a week. Do you want to know the greatest difference between swimming and running? In swimming you can do intervals every practice, even twice a day. Most competitive swim programs have their swimmers do easy intervals in the morning and hard intervals at night. How is this possible? It is because of the absence of the pounding caused in land running, and the therapeutic recovery powers of water surrounding the muscle. I am not saying that you should do all running intervals in the pool, but that you can supplement your land intervals with water intervals.

The water intervals not only allow you to do more work than you can on land, but help you recover from the land "pounding" workout. The water intervals also allow you to continue training even while injured or rehabilitating. This will allow you to keep your fitness level up while you are limited to the pool. I have seen a trend in many runners such that just as their training is going in a direction to truly take them to their personal records (PRs), they get an injury and lose a week or more of training and have to start at the training drawing board all over again. Deep-water running can break this cycle and have your training constantly progressing.

Objective: The idea behind intervals is to go faster (at a higher heart rate) than you can sustain during an entire race for a short period of time. Your heart rate will be at the top of the aerobic range and will actually dip into the anaerobic range at times (see Chapter 8). This causes overloading of the muscles, making them reach a new level after rest.

How it is done: There are a number of ways to do intervals. In the simplest form you could go one minute fast and one minute slow. If you are well versed in land intervals, simply pick a time that would represent the length of the interval you want to simulate and then go hard for that long.

Example: For me, a good track workout starts with a two-mile easy run (approximately sixteen minutes). Then twelve intervals of a quarter mile on the track with a quarter-mile jog/walk between. I go about seventy-five to eighty seconds at a heart rate of 165. Then I go an easy quarter mile (that takes about two minutes), then I do the next quarter-mile interval. After the last interval I do another two-mile cool-down (again approximately sixteen minutes). In the pool I simply start by running easy for about sixteen minutes. I then use my heart-rate monitor to make sure I get my heart rate up to 149 (due to water temperature and increased venous return, heart rate is lowered by 10 percent in the water). I keep a heart rate of 149 for seventy-five seconds, then I go easy (with a heart rate at 120) for two minutes. I repeat this twelve times and finish with a sixteen-minute cool-down. Applying this same logic, you can do longer and even shorter intervals simply by using the length of time of the interval on land and measuring the intensity via heart-rate monitoring. Since there are no miles in the pool, everything is quantified in terms of minutes for distance and duration. Heart rate defines the intensity.

FACT: Your water-running cadence has been proven by researchers at Baylor University to correlate with your heart rate. So, if you increase your cadence, you bring up your heart rate.

Frequency: You can make use of this interval workout much more often in water than on land. You could actually do it every day, although I would not recommend such a routine because of possible mental burnout. Try two a week, one longer interval (half-mile to one-mile equivalents) and one shorter (one-eighth-mile to quarter-mile equivalents). If you are running on land as well, see how one land and one water interval session works. Most athletes find they can actually do more because the water helps so much with recovery.

Fartlek: This should be called random or subjective training. You go hard at random points for a random period of time, then rest for a random period of time. This workout is an interval workout in disguise and should be considered as such. I recommend it for athletes who feel unsure whether they are up to an interval workout or not. Invariably they get into the workout and feel great.

Objective: To do intervals in a different, challenging, and intuitive way.

How it is done: Warm up for ten to fifteen minutes. Next exercise for twenty to thirty minutes, alternating fast and moderate speeds. Vary the duration of the fast and moderate intervals. Follow this by an easy ten- to fifteen-minute cool-down run. Many times it is fun to alternate the effort. Often the workout takes on the form of a ladder. Go fast for one minute, easy for one minute, fast for two minutes, easy for two minutes, fast for three minutes, easy for three minutes—up to as many minutes as you like.

Frequency: This workout is good to do once per week.

In all deep-water workouts, alternate long and short strides.

SUMMARY

We have covered many aspects of deep-water running in this chapter and I hope that you leave with two concepts planted firmly in your mind.

Deep-water running is one of the best activities to prevent injuries and improve your performance if you are a competitor.

If you are not a competing runner, understand that deep-water running has all the benefits of running on land without any of the common drawbacks.

5

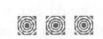

Swimming

What do all the following have in common: stress fractures,
arthritis, anterior cruciate ligament tears, meniscus tears,
plantar fasciitis, neuromas, bumps, and bruises?
Swimmers don't get them!!!!

INTRODUCTION

Despite all the current interest in new ways of working out in the water, swimming is still the most popular. As a matter of fact, swimming is the most popular sport of all—it is estimated that there are sixty-three million swimmers in United States alone. Swimming is popular for good reason. It is a total body workout that works virtually every muscle in the body. The cardiovascular workout from swimming is a great way to stay heart-healthy.

Covering every aspect of swimming would be impossible. So what I will do is give you some up-to-date information to allow you to improve your technique and help you set up a powerful workout program. We will focus on the freestyle stroke (sometimes referred to as the crawl) because it is the most popular and the other three strokes have many similarities. Freestyle is the most popular and most widely used stroke for both competition and fitness. For the interested reader who would like to delve further into swimming, I suggest purchasing the video *Swim Power* and the book *The Essential Swimmer*. Getting someone to videotape you swimming would also be very helpful. Although for all practical purposes swimming is an injury-free activity, make sure you do not cross your arms across the body's midline since this movement can cause swimming's only possible injury: shoulder tendinitis.

You need a certain amount of skill and comfort level to swim, unlike the other forms of exercises in this book. This section is not intended to teach swimming. If you can get across the pool and are not fearful that you will drown, then this section will be helpful to you. If fear of the water is a concern for you, then I suggest you start with some supervised training. A good community swimming class with other people is usually the best way to start to relax in the water. Just make sure the instructor is sensitive to your fears.

There are many developments in technology that have enhanced swimming's development. Underwater cameras have helped coaches dissect exactly what the better swimmers doing that make them so fast. Goggles allow swimmers to stay in the water longer and see the walls better for turning. Electronic timing has made it possible to determine finishing order and times more precisely and to establish accurate records.

It is interesting to note that many swimmers are heading back to the open water to swim. Whether for training, racing, or just plain recreation, the open water has an element of adventure you cannot find in the pool. There is never a problem finding "an open lane" at the beach. There are other elements to consider in open water, such as boats, jetskis, surfers, and creatures. Swimming in protected areas (with a lifeguard on duty) is your smartest option. Triathlon is a growing sport and one of the key elements is the sense of adventure and survival gained by swimming in the open water.

FREESTYLE TECHNIQUE: TIPS WITH DIRECTED DRILLS

In this section I will point out three of the most important aspects of freestyle and suggest some drills to help improve these areas of your technique. Later I will lay out a plan for incorporating the drills into workouts so that you can improve fitness and technique in each workout.

TECHNIQUE

Three of the most important aspects of good freestyle technique are:

1. Long strokes: Long, smooth strokes work best.
2. Bend your elbow before you pull back: Bending your elbow allows you to access the power from your latissimus dorsi and to use a large pulling surface (hand and forearm).
3. Stay on your side as much as possible: This is probably the single most important aspect of swimming technique. This allows you to be

more streamlined, and helps promote a great body position. This will also help make the strokes long.

Certainly there are other aspects to be considered; however, these three form the basis of efficient swimming. The absolute best way to work on them is to do drills each and every practice. Let's examine each aspect and the drills used to guide you to improvement.

Long Strokes: This one makes logical sense. Think about power-racing boats and sailboats. They have long hulls for speed and efficiency. Similarly, swimmers get a longer pull with longer strokes, allowing them to apply force over a longer distance.

There are two movements that determine the length of your stroke:

A. How well you extend your arm forward under the water.

B. How much you rotate on your side as you perform the extension.

The key to extending the arm forward is to slip it in just under the surface of the water and extend forward, keeping the arm just under the surface of the water. Avoid pressing your arm down.

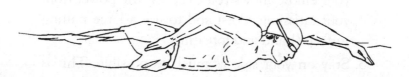

Extending arm

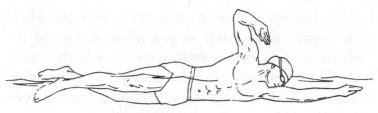

Extending on your side

Rx drills: Two drills helpful for this are single-arm (see page 77) and catch-up (see page 77).

The rotating of your body, referred to as long-axis rotation or body roll, is addressed as the third important aspect of swimming technique.

Bend your elbow before you pull back: When you watch world-class swimmers you may see many different techniques, but one common element is that they all bend the elbow early in the stroke. One of the most common errors we see in our swim clinics is the pressing down of the arm, and a pull with no or little elbow bend. The first change that needs to take place is to lengthen out the stroke as described above, then to bend the elbow before pulling back.

Rx drill: Fist drill (see page 77).

Stay on your side as much as possible: This one is Physics 101. Less frontal area, or drag, with the same amount of propulsive force takes you

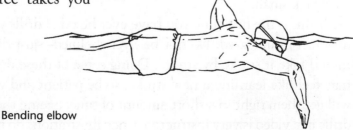

Bending elbow

swimming

75

farther. The key to this one is to try to keep the whole body aligned as one unit as you rotate and avoid the "fishtailing" that comes from rotating only the upper body. The following drills were designed to do just that: Rotate the body in alignment, initiating the roll from your kick and hips.

Rx drills: Kick-on-side drill (page 78), fingertip-drag drill (page 78), kick-on-back drill (page 79), and vertical-kick drill (page 79).

DRILLS: HOW AND WHY

The best way to improve and maintain your freestyle technique is by performing stroke drills. When doing drills it is important that you concentrate on the change you want to make. Going through the motions of the drills is not enough. Instead, you must focus your attention on the desired change; you may be breaking a habit that has been around for a while.

Swimming fins will be of great assistance on all of these drills. Because of the slower and sometimes singular movements, drills are significantly slower than normal swimming. The fins help you maintain speed so that you are not practicing a body position that will be different than your usual one. The best fins are the Zoomer™ fins. They will give you the added speed and allow you to keep your kick small.

If this is the first time you have ever heard of drills you may feel intimidated. Do not be overwhelmed—just dive in and take it stroke by stroke. Doing some of these drills may feel like learning a new stroke, so be patient and you will get them right in a short amount of time. Seeing these drills in a video is very instructive since illustrations do not always help in understanding how they are performed. Drills must be performed with every workout. They serve to remind your nervous system of the way in which you intend to move your body. Drills should be performed after warming up and before cooling down.

Single-arm drill

How to: In this drill you swim with one arm only. There are two separate drills here, left arm only and right arm only. One arm stays out extended in front while the other arm strokes.

What it does: This drill is terrific because it allows you to concentrate on one arm at a time. You can actually watch your arm as you take it through the five phases of the arm cycle.

Catch-up drill

How to: When performing this drill you wait for one hand to enter before pulling with the other. It is like alternating single-arm drills.

What it does: This is an excellent drill in helping you work on your rotation and arm extension. It also helps you work on your rhythm. The rhythm in swimming equals the timing of your pulls, kick, and glide. This is very individual and is perfected by experimentation. This drill is the most helpful in experimenting and feeling relaxed and comfortable in the water.

Fist drill

How to: This drill is performed by swimming the normal freestyle stroke, with the slight change of making a fist with each hand. When you perform this drill, feel the pressure from the water on your forearm. The optimum way to perform this drill is to open your hand in the middle of the lap. Do one and a half lengths and then open the hand immediately. You will realize how powerful it is to have the bent elbow under the water.

What it does: This drill helps maintain a high elbow (underwater), which allows you to employ the powerful muscles of your back for your pull. The reason this drill works is that it forces you to bend your elbow and use your forearm.

Kick-on-side drill

How to: To perform this drill, lie on your side and put your bottom arm out in front of you and your top arm on your side. This is simply the flutter kick performed on your side. To learn this drill do an entire lap on one side; as you get proficient you will want to do six to ten kicks on each side and then alternate sides. This alternating from one side to the other should be a snapping, sharp, total-body movement. Try to initiate the movement by accelerating your kick.

What it does: This drill will help you with your rotation along the long axis and help build endurance in your kick. It forces you to rotate the entire body and not just the torso. You also get to work on kicking the correct way. Kicking with a kickboard is not the way you should kick while swimming; that is a poor way to train your flutter kick.

Fingertip-drag drill

How to: To do this drill you drag your fingertips across the water on the recovery. In order to do this, you need to relax your hand and maintain a high elbow on the recovery. Drop your hand in when it starts to feel heavy. Try to stay on your side for as long as possible as you drag your fingers along the water. The point at which your hand feels heavy will be the correct position for entry.

What it does: This drill helps keep a high elbow on the recovery phase of the arm cycle, keeps your hand from recovering too high and slapping the water, and helps keep you on your side. This drill helps you work on a smooth and clean (no-air) hand entry. It also helps reduce unnecessary tension in your hand during recovery.

Kick-on-back drill

How to: This drill uses a backstroke kick. Simply stated, it is the flutter kick on your back. Alternate one leg coming up (upbeat) with one leg going down (downbeat). As in the freestyle kick, point your toes and move your legs using the upper muscles of your legs, hips, and buttocks. Your hands may be either at your side or stretched out over your head in a streamlined position.

What it does: This drill is helpful in balancing your muscle development. In all forms of physical training, it is always helpful to work muscles in opposing motions.

Vertical-kick drill

How to: You will need the deep end of a pool for this drill. Flutter kick vertically and use your kick to rotate ninety degrees to one side, then use your kick to rotate ninety degrees to the other side. This is a strenuous drill. You will probably be able to do only thirty seconds to one minute at a time. You can go longer as you feel stronger.

What it does: This drill will help you learn to initiate your rotation from your kick while providing one heck of a tough workout.

The best time to "let go" of technique and focus on exertion level is during main sets. The best swimmers in the world perform drills. If you do drills you will be in good company. This is the cerebral part of swimming. You are training your motor neuron pathways and you must visualize the changes before you make them. You may feel awkward at first, but that is a good sign that you are doing something different.

Technique training is an ongoing process and at first it may seem like drudgery, but, in fact, the ongoing process is what makes swimming exciting. You can look forward to always improving, even as you age. How does the phrase "ageless athlete" sound? The majority of masters swimmers swim faster as they age. Of course there is a physical limit (it's older than you think). Are these older athletes stronger? Sometimes. Usually they are smarter. Allow yourself to get fascinated by this idea. Read books and magazines, watch videos, and whenever possible watch a swim meet. Better yet, enter one!

SWIMMING AIDS AND EQUIPMENT

The essentials for swimming are a bathing suit (no baggies or bikinis, please!) and goggles. A bathing cap is helpful if your hair has any length to it at all. Fins are great for drills and working the legs extra-hard. I recommend Zoomers™, which are a small swim fin. Pull buoys are helpful for simulating swimming with a wetsuit and for those days when the legs need total rest. For the vast majority of swimmers, paddles do more harm (in the form of shoulder problems) than good and should be avoided. Kickboards are fun to use while you are socializing and are good for working the legs; however, they do not promote long-axis rotation. For that reason, anyone serious about improving swimming skills should do kick sets by performing the kick-on-the-side drill. The rest of the equipment for swimming falls under the category of "pool toys."

HOW TO PLAN A GREAT SWIMMING WORKOUT

For swimming workouts to be effective they need to have a structure that always involves the following:

- Warm-up
- Stroke Drills
- Main Set(s)
- Stroke Drills
- Cool-down

The most common pools used for swimming are twenty-five-yard or twenty-five-meter pools. The following assumes a twenty-five-yard or -meter pool:

Warm-up: Continuous easy swimming for ten to twenty minutes.

Stroke drills: Two lengths of each; total three-hundred yards.

> **Single-arm drills:** Do one length right arm only, followed by one length left arm only.
>
> **Catch-up drill:** Two lengths.
>
> **First drill:** Two lengths.
>
> **Kick-on-side drill:** Two lengths.
>
> **Fingertip-drag drill:** Two lengths.
>
> **Kick-on-back drill:** Two lengths.
>
> **Vertical-kick drill:** Start at thirty seconds.

Main set: While the choices for main sets in swimming are limitless, these are the basic categories of main sets: long continuous swim, long intervals, and short intervals.

Long Continuous Swim: As the name implies, you swim continuously with no stops. The distance depends on your ability, goals, and the time constraints. Start at a distance that feels comfortable and bump it up as your ability and time allow. Intensity level should be 65 to 85 percent of perceived exertion (PE). The purpose of this set is to build aerobic endurance and psychological confidence.

Long Intervals: This workout consists of doing repeats of three-hundred yards or meters or longer. Rest thirty to sixty seconds between repeats. If I prescribed three five-hundred-yard swims, you would swim five hundred yards, note the time you finish, and push off thirty to sixty seconds later. The length of the swim and number of repeats are dictated by your ability and time. Try to make this main set total one to two thousand yards or meters. As a matter of fact, a routine of three five-hundreds is one of the all-around best main sets. In this set, as with most sets, I recommend swims of descending durations. Swim each one a little faster than the previous one. This type of training works the best since it increases the heart rate slowly over time. I usually recommend perceived exertion to be 70 to 90 percent of maximum. The purpose of this main set is to improve aerobic endurance and to help teach pacing.

Short Intervals: This workout consists of intervals of two hundred yards or meters and less. Rest is fairly short between intervals: fifteen to thirty seconds (for improving aerobic speed, i.e., raising your aerobic threshold) or one to several minutes, providing total recovery (for improving speed). A good example is ten 50s with fifteen seconds' rest. You swim fifty yards, rest fifteen seconds, and repeat ten times. Perceived exertion is 75 to 90 percent of maximum. An example of a speed set would be five 50s with two minutes' (total recovery) rest between intervals. Don't let the two minutes fool you. We are going 90 to 100 percent perceived exertion! There are many other main sets you can do if competition is your goal; seek a coach to help you design sets that will take you to your goals. For the fitness swimmer, be creative with your sets and pay attention to pacing. In swimming, heart-rate training is difficult to maintain, so use either perceived exertion as described above, or check your heart rate at the pool's wall by counting heart beats (index finger at carotid) for six seconds and multiply by ten. For more information on heart-rate monitoring, see Chapter 8.

There are a few main sets to plug in for variety. Adjust the repeat number as needed. The form of these main sets is:

$$R \times L \text{ on } T$$

R: number of repeats, L: length of swim, and T: the time between push-offs (interval time). T is up to you to decide and depends on the set.

Supplemental Sets

    A. The Indicator I: 10 × 100s
    B. The Indicator II: 5 × 200s
    C. The Ladder: 50, 100, 200, 300, 200, 100, 50
    D. Speed: 20 × 25s
    E. Endurance: 5 × 300s

Stroke drills: After the main set(s), you should do one or two drills to bring back good technique lost during harder swimming.

Cool-down: Finally, as with any workout, finish with an easy swim of ten to fifteen minutes.

OFF-STROKES

Many principles of freestyle technique can be applied to the other strokes. Backstroke can be viewed as freestyle on your back. The kick in backstroke is the same kick as in freestyle with a slight change in the ratio of forces exerted from the front and back of the thigh. Butterfly can be viewed as similar to freestyle in that you go through the same pull patterns with your arms. Breaststroke is the most divergent from freestyle technique, but it still has some aspects of freestyle pull. Each of the strokes utilizes the streamlined body position; in each (except the backstroke) you breathe out while your face is in the water; and each calls for that elusive "feel for the water." For the interested reader *The Essential Swimmer* (see Appendix I) has a chapter on the off-strokes, as well as on more advanced freestyle techniques.

6

Water Strength-Training

*Sometimes when I consider what tremendous consequences
come from little things . . . I am tempted to think . . .
there are no little things.* —Bruce Barton

INTRODUCTION

J ust like weight training done on land, strength training can be done in the water with specific movements
and using specific equipment. This leads directly to
the strengthening and toning of muscles. The following
program of shallow and deep-water training is specifically
designed to promote muscle strength and endurance, rather
than the aerobic benefits of aqua aerobics, deep-water running, and swimming.

Just as it is often desirable on land to isolate certain
muscle groups, or work on the flexibility of certain joints
or muscles, this can also be done in the water. The follow-

ing program will strengthen the lower body, abdominals, back, upper body, and even the neck muscles. Many of these areas are overlooked both in our day-to-day activities and in our land workouts. The water provides a wonderful medium that in many ways is superior to that of land-based training. The positive-positive force effect of water training (with an isokinetic resistance force of both the protagonist and antagonist muscles) cuts down on the number of exercises needed, since the resistance of water works the muscle positively in each direction. For example, the quadriceps and hamstrings of the thigh can be worked with the same exercise movement. On land you need two separate exercises to achieve this effect because you are working only against gravity.

This chapter differs from the previous three chapters because I will describe various strengthening exercises and leave it up to you to decide whether to incorporate them into either an aqua-aerobics routine or a water-running warm-up (or cool-down), or to perform them as a separate workout altogether. My suggestion is to incorporate the strengthening exercises into your own water circuit-training program. I am limited in the number of exercises I can describe in this book, but don't let that stop you. You are limited only by your imagination. To help your imagination, see the "Suggested Reading" section in Appendix I. Just remember never to force a joint out of its normal range of motion.

THE EQUIPMENT

The equipment for these activities is important, since it adds both versatility and intensity to your workout program. Almost all work in deep water should be performed while you are wearing a floatation device. This will allow you to focus on the exercise and not on staying afloat.

There are kickboards available that come with handles and act as a workout platform for both the shallow and deep water. I recently used one of these workout boards and was amazed at how much I enjoyed sitting on the board and doing leg extensions. The exercises you can do with this board are virtually limitless.

Another vital and important piece of equipment is a workout station, which gives you the opportunity to hold yourself stable and move specific joints and isolated muscles against the resistance of the water. The key is that it helps you isolate muscle groups during your workout.

The use of equipment in the water allows you to do exercises for the back, abdominals, and upper and lower body to obtain results that are more powerful, controlled, and quantifiable than those you can achieve while exercising freely in the water. Resistive cords and cuffs can be added to many movements to increase your training intensity.

Shallow-water workouts create low impact. This impact is delivered to the feet directly, and since we wear shoes for most of our activities, use of water-aerobics shoes is recommended.

Many of the devices that have been described in the previous chapters can be utilized to improve both the deep- and shallow-water workout. For complete descriptions of this equipment with illustrations, see Chapters 3 and 4.

THE MOVEMENTS

These exercises adapt some aqua-aerobic movements, steal a little bit from the water-running program, and utilize equipment to come up with a few new movements.

While performing these exercises it is always important to realize that you need at least a little space in the pool to yourself. Be careful of those around you. Use your equipment to define your space in the pool, whether it is a tether, a stretch cord, or an exercise board.

In order to build strength it is important to achieve a repetitive workout. After a period of four to five minutes of warm-up, in which you gradually increase your speed and warm-up intensity doing exercises such as deep-water running, you should begin your toning workout.

When working out in shallow water always use your equipment at or below the water's surface. There are two ways to increase the strength-training effect of the water:

1. Increase the speed of your movement

2. Add resistive equipment.

When working out in shallow water be sure to maintain a balanced, controlled posture. Water-aerobics shoes are recommended for all shallow-water workouts. In the deep water it is important to remember that the equipment can be used at the surface or under the water. Whenever using an elastic-resistive cord, always position it at or below the water level on the Water Workout Station™, on a lane-line ring, or on the pool ladder. Be aware of where you attach the cord. Even though using cords is relatively safe, there is the possibility of breakage. No one should stand over the attachment site of your cord.

Be sure to utilize the moves described in the aqua-aerobics chapter (see Chapter 3). Shallow- and deep-water strength training should concentrate on movements that isolate particular muscle groups as opposed to the generalized activity of aqua aerobics. For example, leg curls are an isolated movement, while jumping jacks combine many muscle groups. Generally, do ten to fifteen repetitions of the strengthening exercises in this chapter in each set.

Water Workout-Board Exercises: The Water Workout-Board™ (with handles and louvers) can be used in shallow or deep water. However, I find the workout board most effective in shallow water where I can hold my position in the water to apply more resistance to my muscles.

Here are examples of only a few—but the essential—uses of the workout board. The first three movements are performed in an upright position.

EXERCISE	BRIEF DESCRIPTION
Push-pull	Works the chest (push) and back (pull).
Side-to-side	Works the shoulders, arms, and chest.
Trunk twists	Rotate your body to work the abdominal obliques.

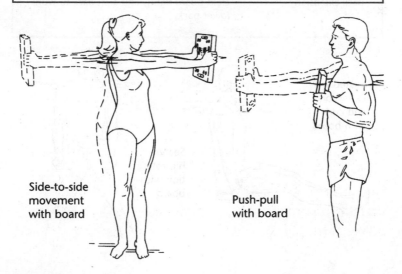

Side-to-side
movement
with board

Push-pull
with board

(For the above three movements, resistance can be adjusted by how much of the board is submerged.)

Sit on the board and hold the side handles for the following three movements. The last movement is done by lying down on the board.

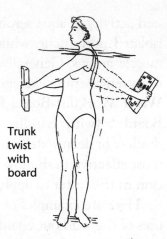

Trunk twist with board

EXERCISE	BRIEF DESCRIPTION
Leg extension/leg curl	Fully extend legs, then return to bent position. Works the quadriceps and hamstrings.
Hip rotation	Do whip/eggbeater kick motion. Works hip internal/ external rotators.
Abdominal crunch	Bring knees to chest to work abdominals.
Back extension	Hold board tightly and arch back to work lower back.

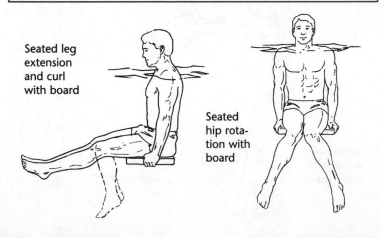

Seated leg extension and curl with board

Seated hip rotation with board

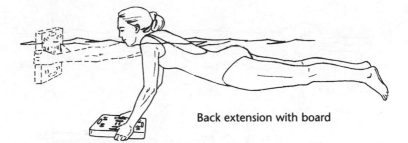

Back extension with board

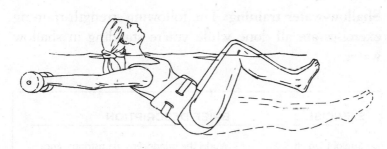

Abdominal curl with hand buoys

Abdominal crunches can also be done in the shallow or deep end utilizing a hand buoy in each hand and drawing the knees toward the chest. Yet another method is done by placing your lower legs over the poolside, keeping your body facing up in the water. Crunch up and hold for ten seconds. Finally, abdominal curls can be done lying back while wearing Flotation Shorts™ and floatation cuffs with elastic-resistive cords on the ankles. The arms can be added to this exercise to work the upper body. We call this movement the "eagle."

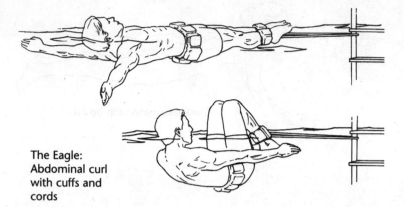

The Eagle:
Abdominal curl
with cuffs and
cords

Shallow-water training: The following strength-training exercises are all done while you're standing in shallow water.

EXERCISE	BRIEF DESCRIPTION
Straight-leg lift	Works the quadriceps, hamstrings, and hip flexors.
Leg curl	Works the hamstrings and quadriceps.
Hip abduction/adduction	Works the abductors (leg out) and adductors (leg in).
Calf raise	Works calf muscles.
Bicep curl (flexion) and triceps (extension)	Positive-positive arm curls.
Trunk twist	Rotate your upper body from side to side to work the lower back muscles.
Back extension	Works the back muscles by arching the back with arms raised or lowered.

(The resistance of all of the above exercises can be increased by the use of cuffs, buoys, and cords.)

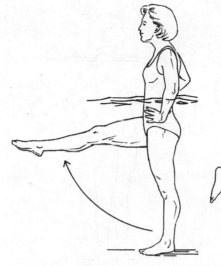

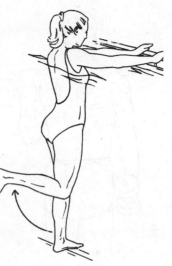

Straight-leg lift in shallow water

Leg curl lift in shallow water

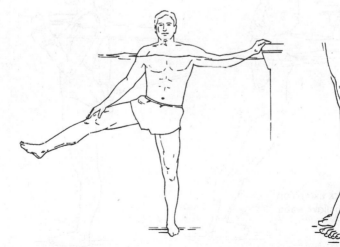

Hip abduction/adduction

Calf raise

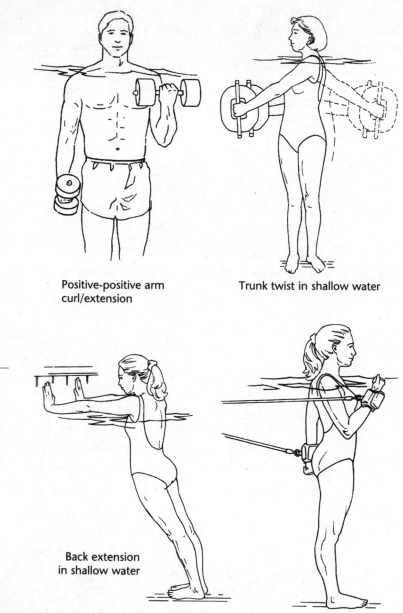

Positive-positive arm
curl/extension

Trunk twist in shallow water

Back extension
in shallow water

Arm curl using resistive cords

The shallow water provides an excellent base for performing upper-extremity exercises. Arm curls to strengthen the biceps and the triceps can be done with dumbbells, swim gloves, or cuffs. The elastic-resistive cords should be worn for a more intense workout. The exercises are done by alternating movements with the hands, first fully extending the arm behind the back and then bringing it forward palm up, and bending toward you, flexing the elbow strongly as you reach toward each shoulder.

Although it does not isolate single muscle groups, cross-country skiing is a tremendous strength-builder when done with elastic-resistive cords on the wrists and ankles. It is an excellent exercise for the lower back, thighs, arms, and buttocks.

Rotator cuff strengthening program: Before we get into specific workout programming, let's look at a very common area of weakness: the rotator cuff. Many people involved in sports such as swimming, golf, volleyball, basketball, bowling, softball, baseball, and all racquet sports, experience shoulder pain. Even if you are injury-free, strengthening the intrinsic muscles of the shoulder is a good insurance policy. Every good therapist knows the exercises that strengthen the rotator cuff and most are performed with free weights or resistive tubing. These movements can be performed in the water with wonderful results. I suggest doing these in neck-deep water, although they could be done in deep water as well. Start with no added resistance and add resistance gloves or cords as you progress. Do two to three sets of ten to fifteen repetitions of each exercise.

On page 99 I describe the five essential shoulder-strengthening movements, which can best be performed while you are standing in neck-deep water.

EXERCISE	BRIEF DESCRIPTION
Seated leg raise	Works hamstrings and quadriceps.
Adduction and abduction	Works hip adductors and abductors.
Lateral trunk swing	Strengthens the torso.
Wide-grip pull-up	Works the latissimus dorsi.
Chin-up	Narrow grip works the biceps and back muscles.
Dip	Works triceps and chest.
Push-up	Hold bench while on stomach and push. Works chest and arms.
Abdominal crunch	Leaning back on bench, pull knees to chest. Works lower abdominals.
Abdominal obliques	Holding hand grips, pull knees up obliquely—first left, then right.

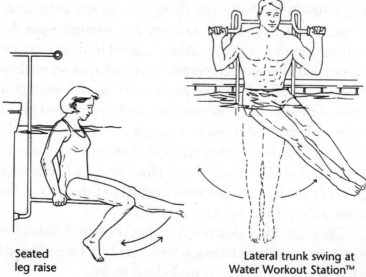

Seated
leg raise

Lateral trunk swing at
Water Workout Station™

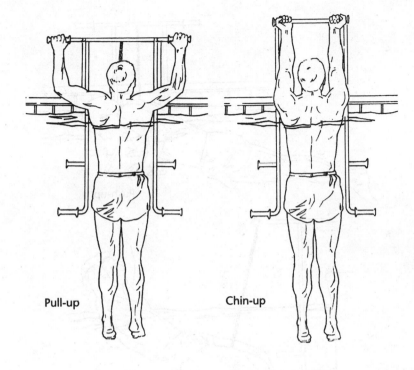

Pull-up

Chin-up

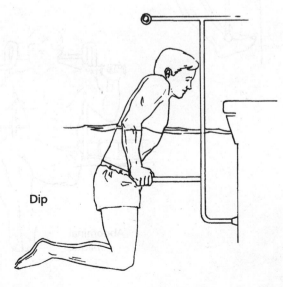

Dip

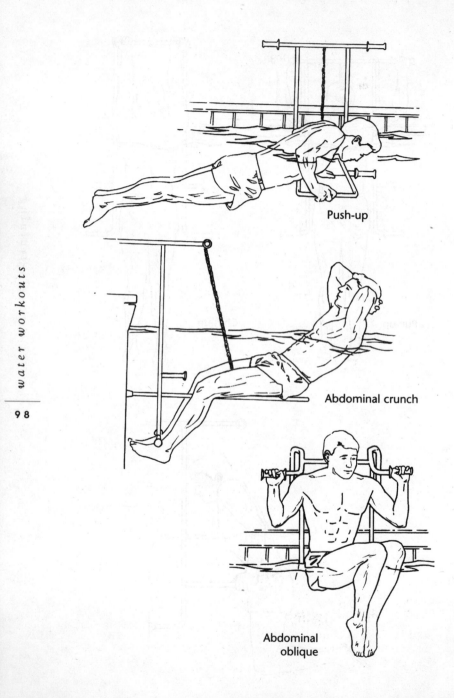

Push-up

Abdominal crunch

Abdominal
oblique

EXERCISE	BRIEF DESCRIPTION
Lateral raise	Raise your arms out to your sides to shoulder height. (See illustration on page 42.)
Posterior raise	Raise your arms behind you as high as you can.
Anterior raise	Raise your arms in front of you to shoulder height.
Shoulder rotations	With your elbows at your side and bent 90°, swing arms in and out.
Shoulder shrug	Shrug your shoulders forward in a circular motion; repeat the shrug in reverse.

Deep-water training: Most deep-water strengthening exercises are best accomplished by utilizing a stationary piece of equipment, such as the Water Workout Station™, pool ladder, or low diving board.

(Remember: If your pool doesn't have a station, try to adapt these exercises to a pool ladder or low diving board.)

While in Flotation Shorts™ or a flotation belt, and with optional use of the elastic-resistive cords, you can do exercises in the deep end that simulate running through tires, and doing jumping jacks while lying on your back.

WORKOUTS: FITNESS AND IMPROVED PERFORMANCE

MUSCLE STRENGTHENING AND TONING

Beginners should focus on ten to fifteen repetitions of each exercise. As you improve, simply add more sets of the same exercise. After you've accomplished two to three sets of an

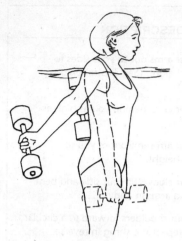
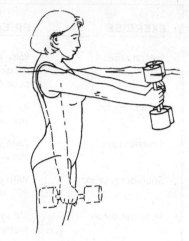

Posterior arm raise   Anterior arm raise

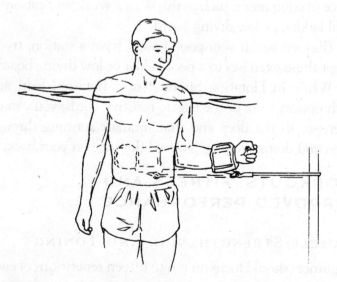

Internal and external shoulder rotation

exercise, use resistive equipment to increase the muscle loading. It is important not to be moving too quickly since you will feel a major burn in your muscle, but a little to moderate burning is good. A major burn represents an increase in lactic acid and turns your exercise into an anaerobic activity.

WATER CIRCUIT-TRAINING

As I mentioned in the Introduction, my suggestion for your shallow- and deep-water training is to do circuit training. The concept of circuit training is to set up a series of different exercises and go from one to the other, in sequence, usually doing ten to thirty repetitions of each exercise. Often the entire series will be repeated two to three times. Circuit training in the water can easily be turned into an aerobic workout by tracking your heart rate. Speed up, or slow down, your movements and rest between exercises, as needed, to stay in your aerobic (fat-burning) zone for a minimum of twenty minutes (see Chapter 8).

The number of repetitions, equipment used, and speed of movement determine intensity. One of the drawbacks of water-based strength training is that resistance against water is less easily measured than the weight of a dumbbell or barbell on land. Therefore, as with aerobic training, a mix of land and water training works best.

Although, as I have said, you can create your own series of exercises, here is a listing of ten essential exercises to get you started. Add to these as you progress. Be careful of your posture and technique as you perform the exercises.

Ten suggested moves for water circuit-training

1. Jogging in place 10–15 minutes (warm-up)
2. Straight-leg lifts
3. Leg curls
4. Hip adductions and abductions
5. Calf raises
6. Biceps curls and triceps extensions
7. Chest flies
8. Trunk twists
9. Abdominal crunches
10. Back extensions

As you exercise you will strengthen muscles, burn calories, relieve the stresses of everyday life, and beat the aging process. Pretty good deal, huh?

SUMMARY

This chapter has given you many movements to strengthen your major muscle groups. It does not include every possible movement. For the reader interested in learning additional exercises, we refer you to Appendix I.

7

◉ ◉ ◉

Performance Enhancement: Sport-Specific Training

Strive for perfection, excellence will come.

INTRODUCTION

Specificity training for sports is using your same muscles in the exact way you do in your sport. The loading of your muscles can be more intense while you are training on water than when you are doing the sport on land. This is the opposite of water strength-training where you isolate muscles to be exercised.

One of the rapidly emerging areas of aquatic exercise in sports is specificity training. By simulating virtually any sport-specific movement in water you gain four benefits: gamma strengthening, the ability to train while injured, biomechanical training, and the "new environment" factor.

Let's look at these benefits in the context of a baseball batter:

1. **Gamma strengthening:** Simply swinging a bat in the water will provide many times more resistance than swinging on land (at least sixty times!).

Batting

2. **Ability to train while injured:** For some injuries the supportive and pressurized nature of water allows movement that would be impossible or damaging on land.

3. **Biomechanical:** The swing of the batter can be analyzed since it is in slow motion due to the viscosity of water. The movement can be analyzed in real time by a coach, or videotaped for closer analysis.

4. **The "new environment factor":** This is the factor that comes into play when an athlete is placed in a new and completely unfamiliar environment and is asked to cope. The athlete is unable to cheat and must function with mechanical correctness in the water. In this situation one cannot fall back on unique strength skills sometimes used on land to overcome a weakness or

deficiency in performing a sport. This is also a renewal training factor.

FACT: Kate McMahon of the New Haven Medical Center has worked with members of the Dallas Cowboys football team in the water to improve specific strength and agility skills. She recommends the "new environment factor" of water to improve performance and coordination for football players.

FACT: A professional baseball pitcher who suffered from severe tendinitis of the rotator cuff was treated in my office. He progressed through a program of flexibility, strength training, and aquatic therapy. A program of pitching in water up to the chin, with and without elastic-resistive cords was implemented. He returned after water training to a position with the Kansas City Royals.

From the example above, you are probably already visualizing swinging racquets, boxing, kicking field goals, etc. One other neat advantage of specificity training is that it takes place in new surroundings—often breathing fresh enthusiasm into the athlete. While you are in the water doing your sport-specific training, take advantage of the opportunity to use some of the other training methods explained in this book. They will also enhance your performance.

FACT: Olympic figure skater Nancy Kerrigan rehabilitated her knee and thigh injury in the water. She now uses an Aquatrend Water Workout Station™ to train. She also does figure-skating sport-specific maneuvers and jumps without risk of injury in the water.

This is a common sequence of events with athletes. They are first introduced to water workouts as the result of an injury, then continue training in the water once they realize the sport-specific benefits.

A classic example of sport-specific water training is the effort our U.S. Olympic runners have undertaken for 1995–1996. A number of these runners have spent many months at the Houston International Running Center with David Brennan, Assistant Professor of Physical Medicine and Rehabilitation in the Baylor College of Medicine.

FACT: David Brennan has devised a program of running in the water for our U.S. Olympic track athletes, with sport-specific training methods in mind. He teaches cadence and proper biomechanics by using underwater cameras and putting headphones with a metronome on every athlete. By gamma-training these runners, he enhances their running performance. Through the use of sport-specific water training, athletes can enhance their track running on land by achieving a greater range of joint motion, improving running biomechanics, and increasing their running pace (increasing cadence).

David Brennan has coined the term "supracadence" to describe the training effect water has on running athletes. He recommends either keeping track of the cadence yourself, an "intrinsic workout," or letting a recorded metronome set up a pace through the use of headphones.

THE EQUIPMENT

The equipment for sport-specific training involves many of the pieces of equipment described in Chapters 3 and 4. Get used to finding a wet baseball bat, tennis racquet, or golf club. I recommend that you use your oldest sports equipment, or equipment that you won't necessarily want to use on land again. Be sure to wash all equipment before using it in the pool.

The use of equipment in sport-specific training is simply to help simulate the movement. Performance can be improved with increased strength, increased endurance, improved technique, and even improved eye-hand coordination. As you go through the motion slower than usual, you can make micro-adjustments.

FACT: Robert Forster, P.T., recommends tethered water-running interval training for track athletes. He has trained three-time Olympic gold medalist Jackie Joyner-Kersee in the water on a tether attached to a floatation device as a regular part of her training program.

There are many examples of sport-specific water-training activities that require no equipment. My work with professional boxers is one example. Generally, they prefer not to use any equipment at all, but when they do use it, they choose hand buoys, resistive gloves, or cuffs with resistive cords in performing their workouts.

FACT: Mohammed Ali and Rocky Marciano routinely trained in the water, doing deep-water boxing exercises as part of their workouts. Their professional records are a testament to the success of boxing in water, either with or without gloves, to improve speed and agility.

Boxing

THE MOVEMENTS

To enhance performance while doing a sport-specific activity, the movement must be biomechanically precise. Because of this requirement, I recommend that you initially work with a coach or a training partner. This coach or training partner can stand above the water, or with you in the water, and watch your technique. This observation is tremendously important in determining the proper biomechanics of your sport activity and the accuracy of your simulation of the movement.

FACT: The U.S. Olympic Track Program uses both underwater windows and a video-camera setup to allow coaches to advise the athletes on specific biomechanical changes in their running. The coaches find that water training helps them do their job better.

Because a training session in water can be seen so clearly, it is an advantage to strength-and-conditioning coaches to use water for sport-specific training. In this way, the athlete can be seen side-by-side with other runners and very close up by the coach. By the use of tethers or elastic-resistive cords, the coach can watch your particular style and technique, and be close by to give immediate feedback.

Tennis anyone? Another form of sport-specific training is the elite tennis player. Tennis racquets are getting wet as players work on their forehand and backhand. These wet racquets help the athletes strengthen the specific muscles they use in tennis, toward the goal of gaining both a competitive edge and enhanced overall performance. You can work on your stroke, on overall conditioning, and on improving your speed in pivoting and cutting. To practice serving you would need to be weighted in deep water and attached to a breathing system—do not attempt this at home or on your own.

I hope your golf club is waterproof since golf clubs are now being used in the water. Clubs are best used in the deep end where there is a lot of room and no chance of hitting the bottom of the pool. Some golfers chop their clubs in half to work in the shallow end. The golf coach can work on a combination of body movements in slow motion, and then speed them up while observing all parts of the swing and follow-through at poolside. This is an excellent method to work on mechanics as well as strengthening.

FACT: Nine-time Olympic gold medalist Carl Lewis enhanced his balance and stance skills for sprinting events by performing balancing exercises in shallow water against a water flume (a forced-water jet) at the Houston International Running Center. These exercises helped him qualify for his fifth Olympic games.

Other examples of sport-specific activities include: hockey players simulating shooting and skating; soccer goalies safely performing kicks and defensive leaping, diving, and jumping; martial arts athletes practicing kicks and jumps; and gymnasts practicing flips and spins over the surface of the water without having to worry about falling on a hard turf or floor and risking injury. Basketball players are able to pass, drive, shoot, rebound, and jump without landing on a hard surface. Any player in a ball-related sport can practice throwing and catching without the risk of impact and injury. They also avoid the curse of overtraining.

FACT: Kevin McHale, former Boston Celtics star, regularly performed water exercises with a sore foot. He also did sport-specific agility and passing drills in deep water.

After your initial work with a coach or training partner I recommend that you continue on your own for a period of time. It is important to have variety in your workout. You should include an aerobic workout and a running workout with your sport-specific training.

WORKOUTS: FITNESS AND SPORT-SPECIFIC TRAINING

It would be rather redundant to list workouts for all the different sports that can be simulated in the water. Here is a general sport-specific training workout.

Sport-specific training workout: Warm up with ten to fifteen minutes of water running or water aerobics. For the next ten to fifteen minutes go through your sports movement slowly, working on the mechanics and taking advantage of the slower speed in the water to make fine adjustments to technique. Increase the speed of the movement and do several thirty-second repeated sets of the movement with thirty-second rests. Try to continue sets for ten to fifteen minutes. This will build endurance and strength. If possible, once muscles have strengthened, attach a resistive cord to equipment and continue the movement to get a gamma loading for increased strength. Cool down for ten to fifteen minutes with water running or water aerobics.

8

◉ ◉ ◉

Training Supplement

Sometimes in life you get a second chance to turn things around; this is one of them.

HEART-RATE MONITORING

The heart-rate monitor is indispensable to the effectiveness of your training program. The American College of Sports Medicine has defined fitness in terms relating to heart rate. This sport-research organization has recommended that a fitness activity be an aerobic exercise (one that keeps your heart rate at 65 to 85 percent of your maximal heart rate) done for at least twenty minutes, three times per week. Simply put, if you don't exercise in an aerobic range, you're not gaining maximum fitness benefits. Five years ago I really had to drill this into the minds of my clients. Lately, more and more people are realizing the benefits of using a heart-rate monitor. Remember, heart rate is the key to exercise level. If you decide not to use a heart-rate monitor, you can take your pulse manually by pressing your index finger on your carotid artery (on the side of your neck, behind your windpipe, and a hand's breadth below your ear) and counting the beats for six seconds. For example, if you count a pulse of twelve for six seconds you then multiply that number by ten and get the beats per minute (BPM); your heart rate is thus 120 BPM. This kind of measurement will only give you an estimate of your heart rate at that instant, since the resultant heart rate can be off by as much as 20 percent! Not to mention the fact that you need to stop or slow down your exercise to take the pulse.

Although there are a few different types of monitors on the market, you should not waste your time with any that are not labeled "ECG accurate." As of yet, no one has come up with a monitor that is accurate without utilizing a chest strap (transmitter) and wristwatch (receiver). The strap fits both men and women and feels a little cumbersome at first, but after a few sessions you will not even notice it. The transmission is wireless so the watch can be placed anywhere as long as it is close enough to receive the signal (usually within three feet). There are several companies that make monitors; Polar Corporation is the most established. The prices vary according to what features you desire. I recommend getting one with a chronograph so you can avoid needing two watches when you work out (see Appendix IV).

It is very easy to fool yourself into thinking you are working out at the proper intensity when, in fact, you may be exercising way below the proper level and not achieving your workout goals. Worse yet is the fitness exerciser who is working *above* the proper level—which can be dangerous! The monitor is a great way to take the guesswork out of your training. Models range in price from under $100.00 to over $300.00 for a model that will download to a personal computer. Whatever monitor you purchase, be sure it is waterproof.

The feedback from a heart-rate monitor is useful in any aerobic activity. Our fitness clients find them very helpful not only in keeping the workout honest, but in providing a welcome distraction from the boredom of some aerobic activities.

Now that you know that you need a monitor and that you should try to stay within your target range, how do you figure out what that range is?

There are different ways to define target range although many amount to the same thing. What follows is a fairly simple, straightforward way to calculate and define three broad ranges of heart zones—anaerobic, aerobic, and sub-aerobic. All of these are defined as a percentage of your individual maximum heart rate; therefore these ranges are different for every individual.

Your maximum heart rate is the fastest rate at which your heart can pump. There are two ways to determine this: by testing or by an equation. The equation method, while simple, is inaccurate and at best only gives you a ballpark figure. The equation is: 220 − your age = age-predicted maximum heart rate (MHR).

There are even qualifiers that try for greater accuracy, such as using 226 for women in place of the 220 used for men. Another method is to subtract your resting pulse before taking a percentage and then adding it back in. Instead of messing around with this fictitious "average" formula, get a stress test conducted by a doctor or another professional. To get the most accurate results you should take these tests while performing your usual activity of choice.

FACT: One of my favorite training partners, Ronnie Schuler (a top age-group triathlete), is over twenty years my senior. We frequently cycle together on training rides. His age-predicted maximum heart rate is 165; mine is 185. His actual heart rate is 181, mine is 174. This is very, very common since the formula again is for a fictitious average person. There are other factors besides age that determine maximum heart rate such as genetics, heart size, and efficiency.

TARGET RANGE (YOUR GOAL OF AEROBIC TRAINING)

Your goal is to stay in the aerobic range because it is the fat-burning zone (the fuel source of choice for both athletes and nonathletes). It is also the best range for exercising your heart and improving your overall and sports fitness. Letting your heart rate go out of target range for more than a couple of minutes greatly reduces the effectiveness of your training. Oddly enough, the target range of most training activities is the same for both athletes and nonathletes because weight-loss athletes, competitive athletes, and fitness athletes all need to promote fat burning.

The exceptions to the rule that you should stay in your heart-rate range are competitive athletes who are sprinters and recreational athletes who engage in quick start-and-stop sports like tennis and basketball. Yet even if these sports are on your list, you still need to do most of your training in the aerobic range in order to build endurance.

Anaerobic training makes up a small percentage of the week's total, and can be skipped altogether if you have no interest in competition or quick, start-and-stop sports.

The following percentages work well for most individuals: anaerobic 80 to 100 percent, aerobic 65 to 85 percent, sub-aerobic below 60 percent. Notice the 5 percent overlap between aerobic and anaerobic training. That indicates the lines are blurred and are defined only by a maximal test. The point when a person switches from aerobic to anaerobic training is called threshold heart rate (HRthr). Your HRthr moves up as you get more fit. The Conconi test is an accurate way to find both HRthr and maximum heart rate. It is a graph of heart rate versus speed (intensity); where the curve bends the HRthr. The aerobic range is five to fifteen beats below that. See Appendix I for suggested reading. It is important to note that heart rates tested in water are 10 percent lower than those tested on land!

Having shot holes in the age-predicted formula and introduced the high-tech method of testing, let's look at two useful and more simple options to find out if you are training in your aerobic range. The "talk test" works great and is more accurate than the age-predicted formula. The test is simply this: Train with a partner and keep up a conversation. If you can barely get out one-word sentences, chances are you are anaerobic. If, on the other hand, you can speak long sentences as you would while sitting at a café, then you are probably sub-aerobic. If your conversation is slightly staccato but you can still converse in sentences (even if shorter than usual), you are probably in your aerobic range 90 percent of your training time.

The other simple way is by using perceived exertion (PE). There are a number of ways to describe PE, as a scale of either one to ten or one to eighteen, or as some percentage of a perceived maximum. Correlating a perceived exertion that is scaled from one to ten during a talk test gives you two indicators for checking your aerobic range.

With all said and done, don't get too crazy about your heart rate and be sure to stay away from both all-out exertion and too low an intensity level. Shoot for a level that taxes you a little, but that you feel comfortable maintaining for twenty to sixty minutes. The American College of Sports Medicine recommends exercising aerobically three to five times a week for the fitness athlete.

FLEXIBILITY

Flexibility is an often-overlooked aspect of fitness and performance. Through the course of normal living, our muscles shorten and, as we age, we naturally lose range of motion little by little. We can also lose range of motion from injuries and overuse. When you notice someone exuding health and youth, flexibility is at the core of what you see. Someone hunched over and taking small steps (basically, someone who is inflexible) does not look, act, or feel vibrant and healthy. The good news is that flexibility and, hence, range of motion, can be restored and improved by stretching.

This chapter will serve as a practical *introduction* to land-based stretching, a subject that should be studied further. (See Appendix I, "Suggested Reading.") One tremendous aspect of training in the water is that it is naturally very conducive to stretching, preventing the tightening of muscles found in almost all other forms of exercise. It is, however, limited in terms of isolating muscles and determining which parts of your body need extra flexibility.

My flexibility study and training led me to meet and work with Aaron Mattes, who has pioneered Active Isolated (AI) stretching. I have found his methods more useful, effective, and enjoyable than all other forms of stretching. He has written an excellent book, which I recommend, entitled *Active and Assistive Isolated Stretching* (see Appendix I). The book expounds a philosophy that includes methods for stretching the entire body.

Training in Aaron Mattes' clinic, I saw miracles daily! He carefully blends flexibility and strength work.

FACT: The ability to achieve twenty to thirty degrees of spinal correction is very common for those scoliosis patients willing to follow Aaron Mattes' program of stretching and strengthening. He advocates early intervention, and states that if tended to early enough, some scoliosis can be totally corrected.

Water work is a form of exercise and therapy commonly recommended by Aaron Mattes. He says: "Water exercise is very valuable for pre- and post-op. It is good for hip and back exercises and helps athletes build stamina and become more explosive. Athletes are limited to the number of jumps they can do on land, but not in the water."

Exercise physiologists and researchers have learned a great deal about muscle and tendon stretching in the past few years. The following is a very simplified explanation of how our knowledge has progressed from ballistic stretching, to static stretching, to Active Isolated stretching.

Ballistic stretching means doing jerking movements to go beyond a certain point in the stretch. This stretching has all but been abandoned since it puts tremendous stress on muscles and tendons and can cause injury. Static stretching, which has enjoyed great popularity, is a gentler approach: You slowly go beyond your "comfortable" stretch and hold it for twenty, thirty, sixty seconds or longer. Although this method is popular, it ignores a very basic principle of muscle physiology: the stretch reflex. The body responds to static stretching (in approximately two seconds) by protectively contracting the very muscle you are attempting to stretch, so you end up engaging in a form of tug-of-war.

Active Isolated stretching has three great advantages inherent in its principles:

1. As you stretch the targeted muscle(s), you contract the opposing muscle(s); this action has the physiological effect of relaxing the muscle(s) you desire to stretch.

2. You hold the stretch for only two seconds, thereby avoiding the stretch reflex.

3. You repeat the movement eight to ten times, allowing you to go farther with each repetition. This also has the effect of bathing the muscles in fresh blood. When employed properly, this method has a marked massaging effect on the muscle-tendon unit and, as a result of the influx of fresh blood (nutrients), speeds healing and recovery.

I recommend concentrating on breathing out through the stretch. This kind of breathing allows AI stretching to be as effective as—or more effective than—a deep massage given for recovery from muscle injury.

Doing Active Isolated stretching in conjunction with your water workouts will give you unbelievable flexibility. For best results, do a quick, light warm-up stretch first and then a more progressive session after your workout.

STRENGTH

A strength-training program should address the entire body. This can be done both by isolating muscle groups and by working them in combinations. I can tell you, from my experience as a personal trainer, that strength training is one of the cornerstones of health. It helps to prevent osteoporosis, increase confidence, and improve performance. Strength training is for people of all ages, especially the older population. Strength training has been proven to be as successful in water as on land—and possibly safer. Children (including young adults who are still growing) should not lift heavy weights, because their bones are still growing. Because of this limitation, the water is an ideal environment for them. Children should concentrate more on strengthening exercises that use their body weight and the resistance of water. Some examples are: push-ups, pull-ups, and dips.

To increase strength in muscles you need to work them two to three times per week. Do one to three sets of ten to fifteen repetitions of each exercise. When you can easily achieve fifteen repetitions in good form, you should increase your resistance by 5 to 10 percent on land, or add a cuff or buoy in the water. For exercises that use your own weight combined with water resistance (such as exercises on the Water Workout Station™), simply keep increasing repetitions in good form. Good technique is the most important part of strength training. It does not matter how much weight you can lift if you are jerking it and using momentum rather than the specific muscles to be isolated.

SUGGESTED LAND-BASED STRENGTH-TRAINING PROGRAM

First begin with a complete stretching routine, as described in the earlier section on AI stretching.

EXERCISE	MUSCLES	TYPE OF EQUIPMENT
Squats	Gluteals, quads	machine or free weights
Leg extensions	Quadriceps	machine
Leg curls	Hamstrings	machine
Calf raises	Calf group	machine or free weights
Lat pull-downs	Latissimus	machine
Push-ups	Chest	none
Dips	Triceps, deltoids	machine
Pull-ups	Arms, shoulders, back	machine
Shoulder presses	Deltoids	machine or free weights
Biceps curls	Biceps	machine or free weights
Triceps extensions	Triceps	machine or free weights
Abdominal crunches with knees at 90 degrees	Abdominals	none
Reverse sit-ups	Abdominals	none
Lower-back extensions	Erector spinae	none
Trunk twists	Abdominal obliques	none

The following exercises can be done at a gym with free weights and/or machines. If you are unfamiliar with weight training, I recommend the book *Basic Weight Training for Men and Women* (see Appendix I). I highly recommend services of a personal trainer or physical therapist to show you exactly what to do with weight training.

Correct pacing and breathing for all strength training is as follows. During the positive move (lifting or pushing the weight) breathe out on a two-count. During the negative move (bringing the weight back) breathe in on a four-count. The negative movement is where much of the strength is gained.

Whenever possible, use free weights and work limbs separately in order to improve balance, isolate muscle groups (just as you did for flexibility training), and prevent compensation by a stronger side. Keep an exercise log. Alternate hard and easy days to improve your strength training. A good way to get started on a program like this is to join a well-equipped gym and have several sessions with a club fitness trainer to get oriented to the equipment.

NUTRITION

There is certainly no shortage of nutritional information available. Numerous guidebooks and videos line store shelves. With so much information accessible, knowing how to select a healthy diet can be confusing. Not only are there many choices, but individual needs also vary, and food allergies and sensitivities need to be addressed one on one. On top of that, there are many variables and stresses that change the demands of our bodies. No one program or ratio of fat: carbohydrate: protein is optimal for everyone all the time. What follows are some of the guidelines that I have found helpful for myself and for the many clients and athletes with whom I work.

Quality food selection, hydration, and timing are crucial for achieving good health and optimal performance. Some athletes also find supplements beneficial. Each of these topics is discussed in this chapter.

The selection of high-quality foods can enhance athletic competitiveness by providing the fuels needed for energy and for tissue development and repair.

The closer your diet is to whole, unprocessed foods, the better you will feel and perform. And the higher the water content, the better the choice. Fruits and vegetables are key, and it is helpful to juice some of them since this process yields a more concentrated source of vitamins and minerals. Whole-grain cereals and breads should also be emphasized since they provide additional carbohydrate calories to fuel muscle and brain tissue. Staying well hydrated is essential. Refrain from or limit consumption of meat, saturated fats, coffee, alcohol, and refined sugars. You do need some fat for hormone production and for lubrication of the organs. Consume only high-quality fats, such as olive oil, avocado, and other vegetable oils. A little fat (15 to 30 percent) will help you sustain a higher energy level.

Staying well hydrated is at least as important as selecting the correct foods. Drink plenty of fluids, especially water. Water makes up the largest percentage of the body and is involved in almost all processes, such as stabilizing body temperature, transporting nutrients, and converting fat to a usable energy source. Inadequate fluid intake reduces your ability to perform these tasks and limits your ability to achieve your potential.

Supplements can be helpful, but they should be pre-scribed by an experienced professional. Some personal trainers are well trained in nutrition, but a better choice is a sports nutritionist or chiropractor. To avoid possible bias, try to work with someone who does not sell vita-mins. My personal recommendation for supplements is a powdered multiple vitamin/mineral combo. The powder mixed with juice provides the most effective way to take supplements. Your body does not have to break down a pill and you have the additional fluid intake. All One Powder™ is the best product I have seen. In addition, mineral supplementation is important. See Appendix IV for information.

When you eat can be as important as what you eat. Try to eat a hearty breakfast. If working out is the first thing in your schedule, then plan to eat as soon after as possible. Try breaking up meals and doing what animals do: graze. Snacking on fruits and vegetables between meals is a great way to get vitamins, minerals, and energy. Try to eat light at dinner and not too late. Eating a heavy dinner at a late hour is one of the worst diet habits. As your body is winding down and preparing to rest, it gets overloaded with the hard work of digesting a big meal. For those trying to lose weight, eating late is "diet suicide": More calories are stored as fat if consumed at night rather than earlier in the day.

Keep healthy snacks, such as dried fruits, bottled water, nuts, seeds, and energy bars, handy in case you have to delay or miss a meal. Do not skip meals purposely.

Proper nutrition is a personal, subjective concept. Try some of the ideas here. Read some of the books listed. Find people who are getting results. Then listen to your own body and mind and develop eating habits that serve you best.

BREATHING

Breathing is one of those automatic functions we take for granted. Each breath in brings oxygen and each breath out expels toxins. With each breath we are "feeding" ourselves the oxygen we need to sustain life and health. The more efficiently we breathe, the more efficiently we transfer oxygen to our cells, and the more completely we remove waste products. Many health experts feel that one of the best things you can do for your health is to take ten slow, deep breaths a day. You should take more time to breathe out, making sure to exhale fully.

Getting control of your breathing is always important because it gets you in control of your body. To do this you should focus on the exhalation. You can use breath control to calm yourself down any time and any place. Your inhalation is automatic. The fight-or-flight syndrome brings on quick inhalations, setting off a number of processes that are helpful in emergency situations, such as when you find a car racing toward you and you need every bit of adrenalin and alertness to "flight"-run out of danger. However, panting and taking short, quick breaths is not advantageous in most situations. So focus on long, slow exhalations. See Appendix I for the book *Breathplay*.

THE MIND CONNECTION

The mind (or brain) controls everything we do. It never ceases to amaze me how we humans can get so wrapped up in our bodies: working out; going to the hair salon; getting waxed, buffed, and toned; providing ourselves with great (and often expensive) nutrition; taking vitamins and herbs; seeing doctors and therapists—often neglecting the organ that controls everything! The mind.

Regular fitness activities, particularly those done in the water, can provide a tremendous mental edge. Many people who might not otherwise be able to exercise applaud the benefits of water workouts. It is beyond the scope of this book to get into any great detail on how best to approach tending to the mind. The subject is not nearly as straightforward as fitness. The health of your mind is a very individual issue and usually touches on spiritual as well as psychological issues. Activities such as yoga, meditation, prayer groups, psychotherapy, "real" vacations, and meaningful relationships are all examples of activities that "feed" the mind. Your brain can take you wherever you want to go; feed it well!

Suggested Reading

Active and Assistive Isolated Stretching by Aaron Mattes. Published by Aaron Mattes, 2828 Clark Road, Sarasota, FL 34231, 1996. This is a pioneering book on flexibility and strength training. Aaron's clinic in Florida is a place where injuries are treated and athletes are trained for peak performance.

Aqua Aerobics: A Scientific Approach by Tom Kinder and Julie See, E. Bowers Publishing, Dubuque, IA, 1992. This book describes basic information and exercise principals for an aquatic aerobic program. Sample programs and specialty programs for older adult exercisers are included.

Basic Weight Training for Men and Women by Thomas Fahey (Second Edition), Mayfield Publishers, Mountain View, CA, 1994. A good book to show you the various ways to work your muscles using free weights and machines.

The Breath Play™ Approach to Whole Life Fitness by Ian Jackson, Doubleday and Company, Garden City, NY, 1995. A step-by-step guide to more powerful and efficient breathing.

The Complete Waterpower Workout Book by Lynda Huey and Robert Forster, P.T., Random House, New York, NY, 1993. Program outlines with illustrations for water fitness-workouts, with an emphasis on injury prevention and healing.

Eat to Win and Eat to Succeed by Robert Haas, M.D., Signet, New York, NY, 1983, 1986. Some good tips on nutrition and the athlete. A nice approach to achieving balance in terms of diet.

The Essential Swimmer, by Steve Tarpinian, Lyons & Burford, New York, NY, 1996. In-depth swim techinque.

Nutritional Healing by James and Phyllis Balch, Avery Publishing, Wayne, NJ, 1992. Source for answering all of your technical questions on nutrition.

The Seven Habits of the Highly Successful by Stephen Covey, Fireside Books, New York, NY, 1990. Cutting-edge technology on managing your time and life.

Swimmers' Guide by Haverland and Saunders, ALSA Publishing, Stuart, Fl, 1995. A reference guide for the traveling aquatic exerciser, with pool listings for all cities in the United States.

Water Fitness Over 40 by Ruth Sova, Human Kinetics, Champaign, IL, 1995. A book written especially for the over-forty crowd, which consistently receives more injuries to the joints and muscles than the younger population (they also work *harder* at their exercise program). A number of exercises are outlined to introduce the novice water exerciser to water aerobics and conditioning. In addition, there are exercises for more advanced fitness levels, many of which can be adapted by users younger than forty.

W.E.T. WORKOUT: Water Exercise Techniques to Help You Tone Up and Slim Down Aerobically by Jane Katz, Ed. D., Facts on File, New York, NY, 1985. An illustrated book that lays out a progressive three-month program of water exercises combined with calisthenics and synchronized swimming.

Now that you have *Water Workouts*, give your swimming the one-two punch by utilizing *Swim Power*, the swimming video that will help you visualize all the concepts in this book. Steve Tarpinian spent five years developing this video, and the reviews from coaches and atheletes agree: *Swim Power* will make a major difference in your swimming. Also look for *The Essential Swimmer*, by Steve Tarpinian, available from Lyons & Burford, Publishers.

To order Swim Power, call 1-800-571-1700 or send check or money order for $39.95 plus $5.05 shipping and handling to:

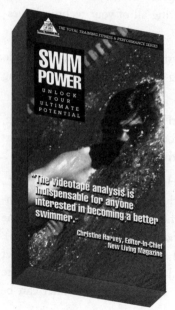

Total Training Inc.
60 East Main St., Dept. WW
West Warwick, RI 02893

For information regarding swim clinics and multisport workshops write to:

Total Training Inc.
78 New Hyde Park Rd.
Franklin Square, NY 11010
or call toll-free 1-800-469-2538
or 1-516-674-4477
email: TTtalk@aol.com

APPENDIX II

Organizations

These organizations are selected for their commitment to aquatic exercise and rehabilitation. They are rated for rehabilitation (R), fitness (F), and emphasis upon aquatic training (T).

American Physical Therapy Association—
Aquatic Section   R
1111 Fairfax Street
Alexandria, VA 22314
Phone: 703-684-2782

American Red Cross   F, T
8111 Gatehouse Road, Sixth Floor
Annadale, VA 22042
Phone: 703-206-7686

Aquatic Exercise Association, Inc.   F
P.O. Box 1609
Nokomis, FL 34274
Phone: 941-486-8600

The Aquatic Therapy and Rehabilitation Institute   R
1032 South Spring Street

Port Washington, WI 53074
Phone: 414-284-3633

The Council for National Cooperation in Aquatics   F
P.O. Box 26268
Indianapolis, IN 46226
Phone: 317-546-5108

Fitness Educators of Older Adults Association   F
759 Chopin Drive, Suite 1
Sunnyvale, CA 94087
Phone: 408-735-9398

The International Health, Racket and Sports Club
Association   F
253 Summer Street
Boston, MA 02110
Phone: 800-228-4772

International Swimming Hall of Fame   F, T
One Hall of Fame Drive
Fort Lauderdale, FL 33316
Phone: 214-637-6282

President's Council on Physical Fitness and Sports   F, T
701 Pennsylvania Avenue, Suite 250
Washington, DC 20004-2608
Phone: 202-272-3421

Resorts and Commercial Recreation Association   F
P.O. Box 12008
New Port Richey, FL 34656-1208
Phone: 813-845-7373

U.S. Water Fitness Association   R, F, T
P.O. Box 3279
Boynton Beach, FL 33424
Phone: 407-732-9908

Publications

The AKWA Letter: Official
Publication of the Aquatic
Exercise Association
P. O. Box 1609
Nokomis, FL 34274
Phone: 941-486-8600

Fitness Swimmer: The Aquatic
Lifestyle Magazine
Rodale Press
Emmaus, PA 18049
Phone: 610-967-8281

Inside Triathlon
Inside Communications
1830 North 55th Street
Boulder, CO 80301
Phone: 303-440-0601

Swim Magazine
Sports Pub, Inc.
228 Nevada Street
El Segundo, CA 90245
Phone: 310-607-9956

Triathlete Magazine
W. Publishing Group, Inc.
121 Second Street
San Francisco, CA 94105
Phone: 415-777-6939

Equipment
Retailers and Catalogs

Aquatic Trends
649 U.S. Highway One, Suite 14
North Palm Beach, FL 33408
Phone: 800-296-5496

Makers of the stainless steel poolside Water Workout Station™

Corflex, Inc.
669 East Industrial Park Drive
Manchester, NH 03109-5625
Phone: 800-426-7353

Makers of the Water Workout Board™, Water Workout (elastic-resistive) Shoes™, water-aerobics shoes, elastic-resistive cords and cuffs, Flotation Shorts™, elastic-resistive swim gloves, Water Horse™, and other aquatic-exercise products.

D.K. Douglas Company, Inc.
299 Bliss Road
Long Meadow, MA 01106
Phone: 800-334-9070

Makers of the Wet-Wrap™ one-size-fits-all upper- and lower-body workout suits for cool water and cool pools.

Excel Sports and Science
450 West Fifth Avenue, Suite 100
Eugene, OR 97401
Phone: 800-484-2454

Makers of the Aqua Jogger™ belt and booties.

Ferno Ille
70 Weil Way
Wilmington, OH 45177
Phone: 513-382-1451

Makers of a portable upright tank for water walking and running.

H_2O Works
585 Slawin Court
Mount Prospect, IL 60056
Phone: 800-426-7353

Retailers of the patented Flotation Shorts™, elastic-resistive workout cuffs, workout gloves, and many types of handheld dumbbells
and paddles.

HydroFit, Inc.
1328 West Second Avenue
Eugene, OR 97402-4127
Phone: 800-346-7292

Retailers of several types of belts, cuffs, and gloves.

Hydrophonics
880 Calle Plano, Unit J
Camarillo, CA 93012
Phone: 800-794-6626

Waterproof and submersible microphones and pool sound systems.

Hydro-Tone Fitness Systems
16691 Gothard Street, Suite M
Huntington Beach, CA 92647
Phone: 800-622-8663

Makers of plastic handheld dumbbells and resistive devices.

J and B Foam Fabricators
111 South Jebavy Drive
P. O. Box 144
Luddington, MI 49431
Phone: 800-621-3626

Makers of foam dumbbells and barbells.

Jo Shel Engineering (Aqua Sound)
P. O. Box 186
Oswego, NY 13126
Phone: 315-343-2857

Wireless microphones for instructors, and sound systems compatible with a pool environment.

Polar Monitor
99 Seaview Boulevard
Port Washington, NY 11050
Phone: 800-742-4478

Makers of a heart-rate monitor with a unisex chest strap and a wrist telemetry unit. A top-of-the-line model allows you to download to your computer.

Sprint-Rothhammer
P. O. Box 3840
San Luis Obsipo, CA 93403-3840
Phone: 800-235-2156

Mail-order sales with a full line of aquatic equipment.

Speedo Authentic Fitness Wear
6040 Bandini
Los Angeles, CA 90040
Phone: 800-547-8770

Mail-order and retail sales of swimsuits, water steps, and a full line of aquatic-exercise apparel.

Strom-Berg Productions
253 Rhodes Court
San Jose, CA 95216

Phone: 800-828-8637

Makers of innovative music for aerobics and water-workout classes and athletes.

Swimex
Route 136, 50 Market Street
Warren, RI 02885
Phone: 800-877-7946

Makers of both club-size and in-home exercise pools with a flume jet powerful enough to allow swimming in place.

U.S.A. Aquatics
120 Country Club Drive, Unit 8
Incline Village, NV 89451
Phone: 800-445-8721

Mail-order sales of TYR, Speed, and Nike, plus an extensive selection of pool and training equipment.

World Wide Aquatics
10 500 University Center Drive, Suite 250
Tampa, FL 33612
Phone: 800-726-1530

Mail-order sales with a full line of swimming equipment, including a section on water training.

Glossary

Abduction: To move your arm or leg away from your body.

Adduction: The opposite of Abduction. To move your arm or leg toward your body. (Hint: The "Add" of Adduction clues you into which direction to go; i.e., adding toward your body.)

Aerobic: A state in which oxygen consumption is increased by improving the respiratory and cardiac organs. This state can be achieved only through various exercises such as swimming, running, and biking.

Anaerobic: A state in which, during heavy exercise, pyruvic acid is released and acts as a hydrogen acceptor, and lactic acid builds up in the tissues.

Antagonist: The muscle that acts in the opposite direction of the muscle you are using (i.e., the quadriceps are the antagonists of the hamstrings).

Arthritis: Injury to the articular cartilage in a joint, leading to pain and inflammation.

Buoyancy: A body's ability to float, or the upward force exerted by a fluid on a body placed in it.

Cadence: Rhythmic, balanced flow of movement, as in marching.

Circuit Training: A series of exercises done sequentially to form a workout routine.

The Eagle: A water-exercise abdominal curl done with elastic-resistive cords on cuffs or shoes.

Elastic-Resistive: The use of a stretchable cord attached to two points (i.e., two shoes or two cuffs) to exercise in a reciprocal fashion. For example, attach a single stretch cord through a ring to both shoes; one side pulls while the other side pushes.

Fartlek: Randomized intervals performed during a workout.

Flotation Shorts™: An exercise buoyancy device that combines floatation with a comfortable pair of shorts that prevents the device from riding up during exercise.

Gamma Loading: Increasing the resistance to a movement many times more than the muscles ordinarily experience.

Gamma Strengthening: An increased strengthening effect due to gamma loading.

Interval Training: A workout that is intense for a period and alternated with easier or rest periods.

The New Environment Factor: The rejuvating effect of a change in the workout program.

Open Water: Any swimming environment other than a pool, such as a lake, pond, or ocean.

Positive-Positive Training: A unique aspect of water strength-training that allows you to work protagonist and antagonist muscles positively with one exercise.

Protagonist: The muscle you are using. It acts in the opposite direction of the antagonist muscle. For example, the triceps are the protagonists of the biceps.

Repeat: Any drill (or length of exercise) that involves doing the same distance or exercise a number of times with brief resting intervals. An individual drill from the set is referred to as a repeat.

Resistance: Force exerted against movement.

Rotator Cuff: The intrinsic muscles in the shoulder that hold it in place.

Set: A group of repititions.

Shallow Water: Any body of water, or part of a swimming pool, where your feet can always touch the bottom.

Shinsplint: Painful inflammation of the tibial and toe extensor muscles caused by repeated minimal traumas.

Supracadence: A word coined by David Brennan of the Houston International Running Center for the increased cadence (stride rate) you can achieve while training in the water.

Target Range: Your personal aerobic heart-rate goal.

Tendon: A tough cord or band of dense, fibrous connective tissue that attaches muscle to bone.

Tendinitis: Inflammation of a tendon. Symptoms can be redness, heat, pain, swelling, and often loss of function.

Tether: A swimming aid that attaches to a swimmer and holds the swimmer in place. Also used to hold deep-water runners in place.

Turbulence: The agitation of the water surrounding a water exerciser, giving a massage effect.

Water Workout Station™: A stainless steel gym that attaches to the edge of a pool and acts as a station for your water training; useful especially for deep-water exercise.

The "Zone": Aerobic heart rate to achieve that puts you in your best fat-burning mode.

Index

water workouts

tennis, 108
tethers, 53
threshold heart rate (HRthr),
115
training frequency, 14
triad, health, 25
turbulence, 7–8

vertical kick, 41, 79
vertical water exercise, 3
vests, floatation, 29, 52

walking, deep-water, 61–2

water
exercise history, 10
physical properties, 6–8
water workouts
benefits, 2–3, 9
effect on land running, 5
myths, 4–6
popularity, 4
weight loss, 6, 19, 22
Wilder, Robert, 54
workout boards, 32
workout stations, 34–35
wrist exercises, 45